A CHRISTIAN LOOK AT

Growing Up Now

YOUR CHANGING BODY
YOUR CHANGING FEELINGS

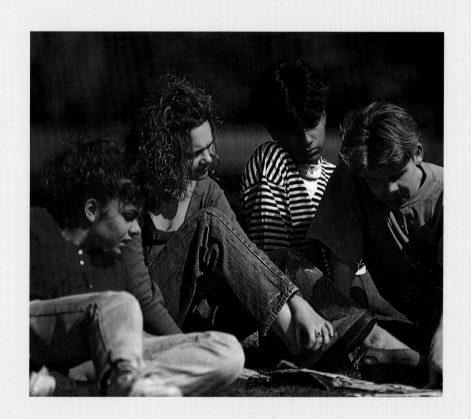

JACK WINGFIELD
MB, BCh, FRCOG

ANGELA WINGFIELD
SRN, SCM, MTD

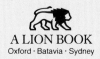

A LION BOOK
Oxford · Batavia · Sydney

Text copyright © 1992 Jack and Angela Wingfield
This illustrated edition copyright © 1992 Lion Publishing

Published by
Lion Publishing Corporation
1705 Hubbard Avenue, Batavia, Illinois 60510, USA
ISBN 0 7459 1537 X

First edition 1992
All rights reserved

Library of Congress Cataloging-in-Publication Data
Wingfield, Jack
    Growing up now: The facts, the feelings, the fun
    Jack and Angela Wingfield
    1. Child development—Juvenile literature
    I. Wingfield, Angela II. Title
    HQ767.9.W56 1992 305.23'1–dc20

Printed and bound in Singapore

Acknowledgments
Bible passage taken from The Holy Bible, New International Version published by the New York International Bible Society.

Photographs
Barnaby's Picture Library, spread 1 (bottom centre) / Richard Gardner, spread 9 (top left); Jeremy Broad, spread 13;
Adam Buchanan, spread 1 (top centre);
Susanna Burton, spread 20 (top);
Cephas/Mick Rock, spreads 1 (bottom right), 10 /Jim Loring, spread 19 (top);
Gordon Coleman, spread 3;
Malvin van Gelderen, spread 9 (bottom left);
Philip Henderson, spread 1 (top left);
Image Bank/Hank Delespinasse, spread 2 (top) /Don King, spread 11 (right);
Camilla Jessel, spread 17 (all);
Eric Marsh, spread 9 (bottom right);
Carrie and Jeremy Pemberton, spread 15 (left)
Network Photographers/Mike Abrahams, spread 19 (bottom);
Iris Poulton, spread 14 (bottom);
Lois Rock, cover (top) and spreads 1 (bottom left), 16;
Nick Rous, spread 9 (top right);
Science Photo Library, cover (centre left) and spread 15 (top and bottom) /John Walsh, spread 5;
Duncan Smith, spread 2 (bottom);
Sterex Academy/Pamela Linforth, spread 8;
Anne Ward, spread 14 (top left and right);
Zefa (UK) Ltd, cover (right and bottom left) and spreads 7, 11 (title page and left), 12 (right), 18, 20 (centre left and bottom)/ Pickerell, spread 20 (centre right) /Sharp Shooter, spread 12 (left).

Illustrations
Diagrams by Oxford Illustrators.
Cartoons by Kim Blundell.

ABOUT THIS BOOK

So much changes when you grow up—your body, your outlook, your relationships—the whole process can seem like a real challenge.

This book is designed to help you meet that challenge. It gives the facts about how your body changes as you grow up, and what these changes are for.

It talks about your feelings, too, to help you understand your changing outlook as you begin to take charge of your own life.

This book is also about the choices you face as you take your place in the world. It raises the questions that you will need to answer in order to get the most out of life. The authors believe that the best guidelines for a happy and purposeful life are those which have been given by the God who made us the way we are.

CONTENTS

Can you remember the day you started school? Just a few years ago, you were looking up to those in the higher classes. How tall they were. How clever. How grown-up.

Now you have reached that stage. You're not yet a grown-up, but you don't want anyone to think of you as just a child.

Perhaps you have already started to grow in all directions! On the other hand, you may be wondering if you will ever change at all. Will you be left behind all your friends, feeling like a baby? What will your body do to you next?

You have ideas of your own now. Once it was fun to be with all the family. Now you want to do things your way. You wish you didn't have to be with them. At least, not all the time.

The fact is, you're growing up in all sorts of ways. Find out about the changes that will happen to you in the next few years, and get ready to deal with them.

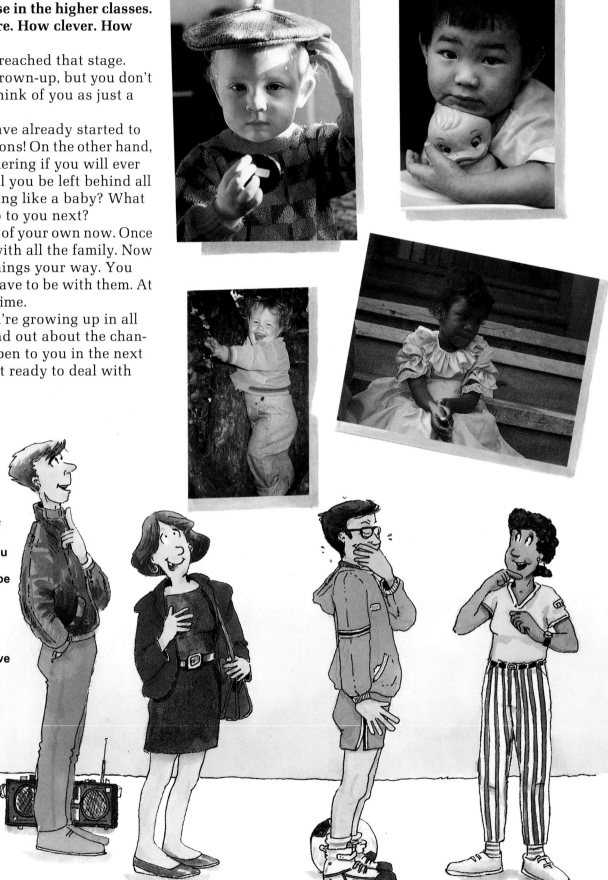

Compare a picture of yourself as a small child with the way you look now. You have grown taller, the shape of your body has changed, and you have a new set of teeth. Your hair may have changed color, and you probably have it cut in a different style—one that you chose!

A PERSONAL ALBUM

Find out as much as you can about how you looked from the time you were a baby up till now. You can ask relatives and friends who knew you at that time, or look at any photos that were taken of you. Draw pictures or borrow photographs to make a personal album of how you have changed.

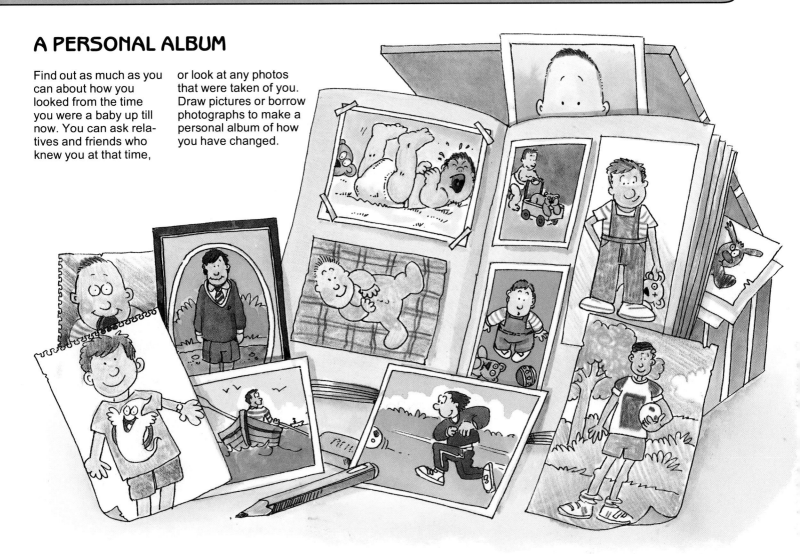

THE SHAPE OF THE FUTURE

What will you look like in a few years' time? Will you still have the same interests that you have now? Will you be free to do what you want? Will you be boring when you're really grown-up? Will you still have fun?

Here are some things that are very likely to happen to you in the next few years:

● Develop a grown-up body.

● Do things away from your family, such as going on vacation with friends.

● Find members of the opposite sex interesting, not silly nor alien.

● Begin thinking about the sort of grown-up you want to be: the type of job you will have, the type of home you will live in, the type of people you will want to have as friends.

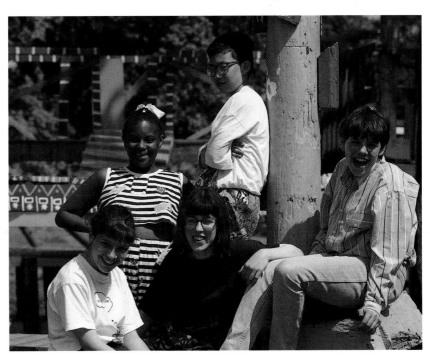

TAKE CARE OF YOURSELF

How much do you know about taking care of yourself? At a time when your body is changing a great deal, it is very important to look after it properly.

You can take at least some responsibility for looking after your body.

Choosing the right foods and getting enough exercise will help you to stay healthy. As a result you will have plenty of energy so you can have lots of fun. Radiant health will help you to look good too.

FOOD

Your body needs food in order to grow. Different foods contain different types of nutrients. You need the right balance of these in order to keep your body healthy. They include protein for growth, fats and carbohydrates for energy, vitamins, and fiber to help your bowels work.

You need to eat a range of foods from these groups in order to get all the nutrients you need.

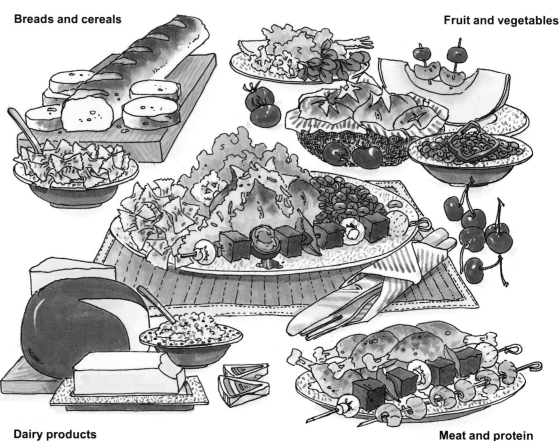

Breads and cereals

Fruit and vegetables

Dairy products

Meat and protein

PACK A HEALTHY LUNCHBOX

If you have to pack a meal for yourself, make sure that it contains food from each of the groups listed above.

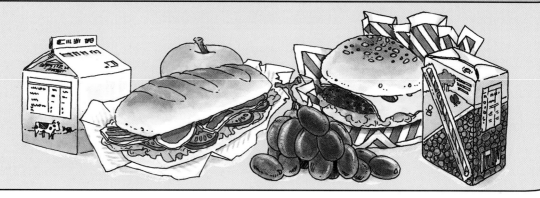

FIT FOR ANYTHING

Exercise should do two things if you want to stay fit. It should make your heart work harder than usual, so that it is able to work strongly all the time. It should also make other muscles work so that they grow strong too. Jogging, swimming and cycling all do this.

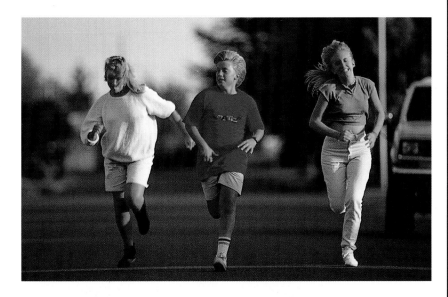

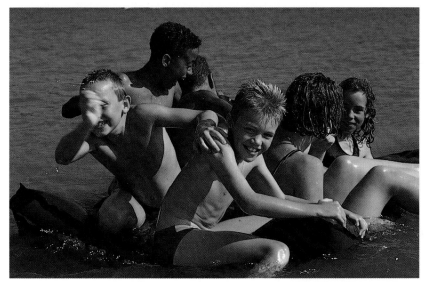

SWEET DREAMS

Rest. How wonderful it is to lie in bed doing nothing. Your body needs enough sleep if it is to work properly. You need around 8 hours' sleep each day.

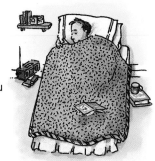

BEAT THE BUGS

Keeping clean is good for you. You avoid many of the kinds of infections that can make you ill, you keep your teeth healthy, and you smell nice.

Wash your hands after going to the toilet

Wash your hands before and after handling food

Brush your teeth every day, morning and evening.

Wash regularly to keep your skin clean

Remove makeup

Your body is going to change quite a bit in the next few years. This is not new. You have been growing ever since you started life inside your mother. Just think: you started life as one cell weighing a tiny fraction of a gram. The average baby weighs 7$\frac{1}{2}$ pounds at birth. How much did you weigh when you were born? How much do you weigh now?

One of the most obvious signs that you are growing up is that you are growing taller.

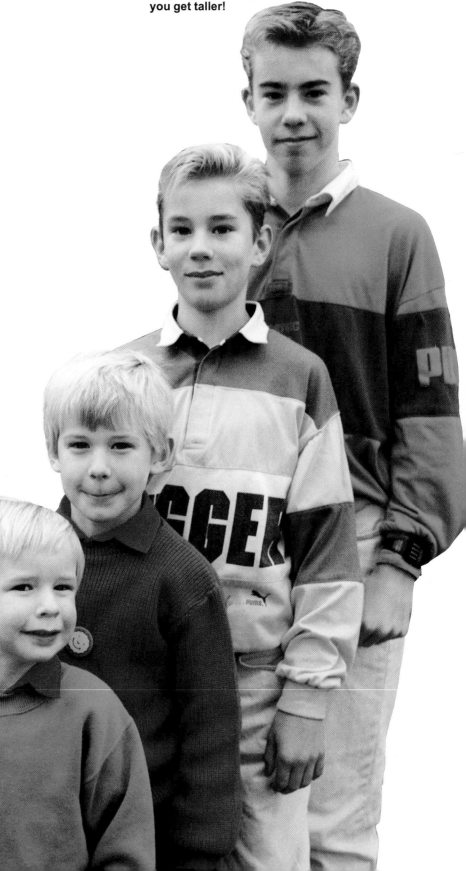

As you grow older, you get taller!

GROWTH SPURTS

Many people have a family measuring chart on a wall or door. They mark their heights and the date.

You may have noticed that babies seem to grow out of their clothes constantly. There have been times when boys and girls around you seem to have grown very fast too. Some people in your class are suddenly almost as tall as the teacher. A period of rapid growth is called a growth spurt.

During the first year of life growth is fast, but after that it slows down. Your height then increases at a fairly steady rate. In the early years, girls are usually slightly shorter than boys of the same age. At the age of 10 they are about the same height.

Girls usually begin their growth spurt earlier than boys. From about the age of 10 to 11 they grow quickly. For a few years they are likely to be taller than boys of the same age. By about 14 this rapid growth will have slowed down, and by the age of 17 most girls will have reached their adult height.

Boys do not begin their growth spurt until they are about 13. Then they catch up the difference in height with the girls and grow a few inches taller. Although their growth rate slows, they will probably keep growing until they are at least 18 or 19 years old.

HAVE YOU NOTICED?

Different parts of the body grow at different rates and also reach their growth spurts at slightly different times.

When you are about 10 you may find that your hands and feet are rather large for the rest of you, and that you keep growing out of your shoes. By the time you are a teenager, your hands and feet will be back in proportion again!

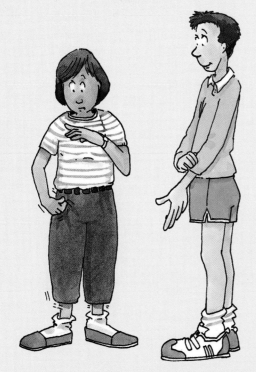

A baby isn't a miniature adult in shape—just look at the size of its head compared with the size of its body. A baby's head is almost as wide as its shoulders and accounts for about a quarter of its total height.

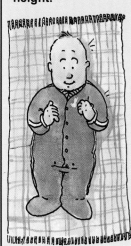

By the time a child is 7 the head is 90 per cent adult size.

By about 10, the brain is more or less adult size.

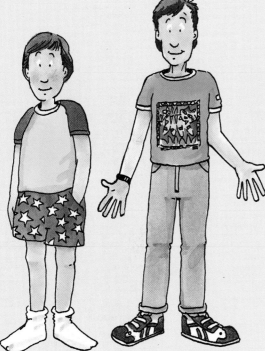

Q *Is it possible to work out how tall I will be when I have finished growing?*

A *Yes, it is. However, to find out properly you would need to have X-rays and special tests. Your best guess is to look at your parents and grandparents—you will have some characteristics from each of them. If they are all short, it is likely that you will be short too.*

Q *All of my younger friends are already taller than me. Am I always going to be short?*

A *Not necessarily. Some people's growth takes a bit longer to get started. Then they grow rapidly and may end up taller than their friends.*

It can be miserable to be a lot smaller than everyone else. If you are worried about your height, go to see your doctor. Occasionally there is a problem that needs attention. In any case, it is nice to check that you have nothing to worry about.

Finally, don't think that height is everything. Differences are all part of God's design for human beings. We are not made to a standard pattern.

DID YOU KNOW?

- People are slightly longer when they are lying down than when they are standing up.
- Your height increases at a faster rate in the spring.
- People gain weight fastest in the autumn.

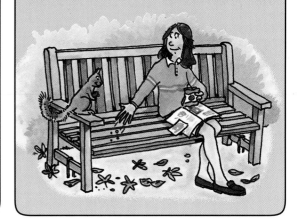

GIRL OR BOY?

Are you a boy or a girl? You have been the sex you are from the moment you were formed. From the minute you were born, people could tell which you were.

The basic difference between the bodies of baby boys and baby girls is the bit between the legs, called the genitals. Boys have penises, girls have a little pad of fat that extends backwards and underneath as two thick folds with a slit between. These outer signs indicate the sex of the baby. Sex indicates what part a person is able to play in reproducing young—whether they can be a mother or a father. Even baby boys have the basic equipment needed for them to father their own babies when their bodies are old enough. Baby girls have the equipment they need to become mothers.

The changes that happen to you as you grow up are closely linked to changes in this equipment. What does it consist of?

GIRLS

The equipment girls have that will enable them to become mothers consists of several parts. There is a place where tiny egg cells develop, a place where these can be fertilized in order to grow, a place where the egg can grow into a baby, and an opening where the baby can come out when it is ready to be born.

View from the front

The Fallopian tubes look rather like out-stretched arms with 'finger ends'. They are about 4 inches long, and they provide a pathway from the ovaries to the uterus. An egg cell, or ovum, is caught in the finger end and travels through to the uterus. The journey takes about a week. It is as the egg cell is travelling in one of these tubes that it can be fertilized by a sperm.

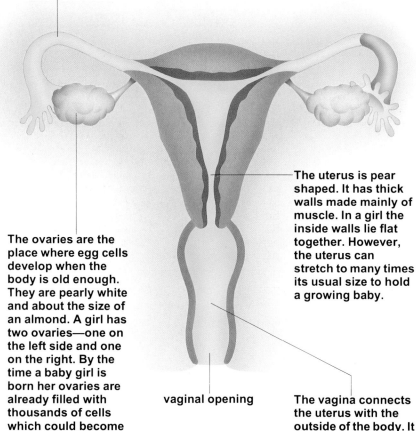

The ovaries are the place where egg cells develop when the body is old enough. They are pearly white and about the size of an almond. A girl has two ovaries—one on the left side and one on the right. By the time a baby girl is born her ovaries are already filled with thousands of cells which could become eggs, although only a few will. An egg cell is called an ovum. The plural of ovum is ova.

vaginal opening

The uterus is pear shaped. It has thick walls made mainly of muscle. In a girl the inside walls lie flat together. However, the uterus can stretch to many times its usual size to hold a growing baby.

The vagina connects the uterus with the outside of the body. It is made of muscle and is arranged in lots of folds so that it can enlarge to let a baby out.

View from below

The vulva is the outside part. At the front is a pad of fat called the mons. Behind are two thick folds which are called lips. Hidden between these two outer lips are thinner and smaller ones. At the front, these form a hood over a small part called the clitoris. These are all very sensitive to touch, and are the parts that grow much larger at puberty. The clitoris is similar to the male penis. Although it remains much smaller than a penis, it is just as sensitive.

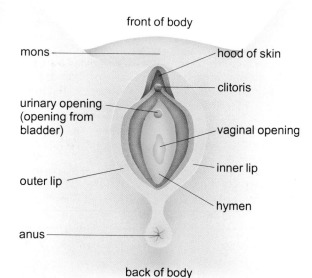

front of body

mons — hood of skin
clitoris
urinary opening (opening from bladder)
vaginal opening
outer lip
inner lip
hymen
anus

back of body

There are two openings between the inner lips. The one in front comes from the bladder. This is where urine comes out. The other is the opening of the vagina. There is a skin called the hymen which in young girls partly or completely closes the entrance to the vagina.

Right at the back is the anus, the exit from the body for waste and undigested food.

4

BOYS

The equipment that boys have is designed to fertilize the egg cells that females produce.

View from the front

View from the side

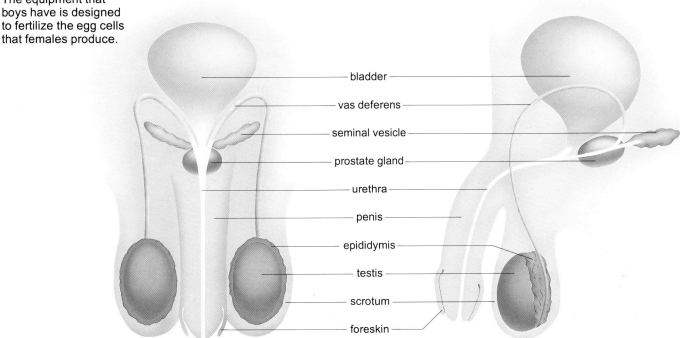

- bladder
- vas deferens
- seminal vesicle
- prostate gland
- urethra
- penis
- epididymis
- testis
- scrotum
- foreskin

There are two testes. These are oval and firm, and are found in a bag of skin called the scrotum, just behind the penis. Inside each there is a mass of very tiny tubes, where sperms are made. Sperms are the tiny cells that can join with egg cells in a special way so that they can grow to make a new human being. Sperms and some fluid travel through the tubes in the testes to the epididymis. Here the sperms mature. Then they travel on to a larger tube called the vas deferens.

The sperms travel through the vas deferens towards the penis, past glands called seminal vesicles and past the prostate gland. These glands make additional fluids which join the sperms as they pass by and help the sperms to move along. This new mixture of fluids and sperms is called semen. Sperms may be stored in the epididymis and in a small part of the seminal vesicles.

The vas deferens links up with the exit from the bladder, called the urethra. Semen can travel through this tube to the exit at the tip of the penis.

Most of the time the penis is small and limp. However, it is made of special tissue that can be pumped up with extra blood so that it becomes firm and erect.

The tip of the penis is normally covered by a piece of skin called the foreskin. In very young boys it is stuck to the end of the penis, but long before puberty it separates and can be rolled back. After puberty, it needs to be rolled back and washed regularly when bathing.

Cirmcumcision is a small operation in which the foreskin over the tip of the penis is removed. Many boys are circumcised when they are babies. Occasionally, men are circumcised later in life, under anesthetic.

Q *Why are the testes in a special bag of skin instead of tucked inside the body?*

A *The special position of the testes keeps them cooler than the rest of the body. This is important, as they don't produce sperms when they are too warm.*

Q *Why do some boys not have two testes in their scrotum?*

A *The testes start to grow inside the body and come down through a channel into the scrotum, usually about one month before birth. Occasionally they get stuck in the little channel and an operation is needed to draw them down into the right place. This is usually arranged at about 10–12 years. The operation might be a bit uncomfortable, but it isn't serious.*

Sometimes before puberty the testes shoot back up into the channel they came from. This can happen particularly in cold weather, or when a doctor examines that area. It isn't a problem, as the testes come back down again just as quickly.

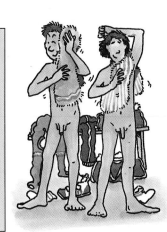

GROWN-UP BODIES

Babies can't have babies! At some stage during the growing-up process, the parts of the body that are there for making babies begin to work. This time is called puberty. When it is complete, the female ovaries regularly produce mature egg cells and the male testes produce sperms. After puberty, the body continues to grow and mature. This time is called adolescence.

WHEN DOES PUBERTY START?

The time when puberty starts is different for boys and girls. Girls' bodies start to develop when they are between 11 and 14 years, and boys' bodies when they are between 13 and 16.

Everyone is different. Some people reach puberty a couple of years earlier, and others start later. There is no need for anyone to worry about whether or not their body will develop in the right way. Eventually, everyone starts puberty.

HOW DOES IT START?

Puberty starts in a small part of the brain called the hypothalamus. When it is mature, or old enough, it starts work and produces special substances called releasing hormones.

At first only small amounts of releasing hormones are produced every two hours or so, and usually when a person is asleep in bed. These releasing hormones awaken the pituitary gland, which is also at the base of the brain. In both boys and girls, the pituitary gland starts to produce higher levels of two hormones, one called follicle stimulating hormone (FSH) and the other called luteinizing hormone (LH).

WHAT ARE HORMONES?

Hormones are part of the body's communication service. They carry messages from one part of the body to another. They are produced in special cells grouped together called endocrine glands. Each hormone carries a different message. Hormones travel in the blood stream.

Not all hormones are related to puberty. Perhaps the best-known hormone is adrenalin. It is produced when something frightens you, and it sends messages to make your heart beat faster and your breathing more efficient. That helps you to run away faster if you need to!

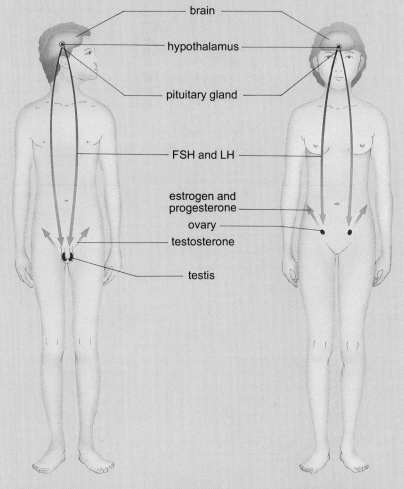

- brain
- hypothalamus
- pituitary gland
- FSH and LH
- estrogen and progesterone
- ovary
- testosterone
- testis

At puberty the differences begin. The female ovaries respond to the hormones from the pituitary gland (FSH and LH) by starting to develop egg cells and by producing large amounts of their own hormones: the main ones are estrogen and progesterone. These cause other parts of the girl's body to grow. All four hormones (two from the pituitary gland, two from the ovaries) work together in bringing about the menstrual cycle.

The male testes respond to their messages from the pituitary gland by starting to produce sperms. The testes also start producing testosterone. This hormone causes other parts of the boy's body to grow.

EGG CELLS

The female ovaries produce a mature egg every 28 days or so. If the mature egg joins with a sperm it is said to be fertilized and will grow into a baby in the uterus. In preparation, the uterus grows a thick lining every time, just in case. If the egg is not fertilized, the lining is shed, along with a little blood. This whole process is called the menstrual cycle, and the slight blood loss is called a period.

SPERM CELLS

The male testes produce sperms, which are shaped like very tiny tadpoles, so small that you need a powerful microscope to see them.

The tail lashes about and this enables the sperm to travel.

The head carries a set of chromosomes, tiny structures which will link up with another set of chromosomes in the egg. The chromosomes contain information about how the fertilized egg will grow.

This photograph shows sperms magnified many times. Each sperm has a head that contains the chromosomes and a tail that the sperm uses to swim.

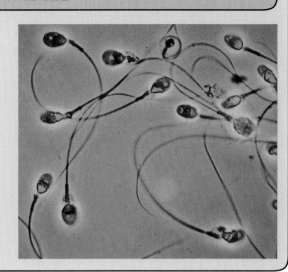

THE MENSTRUAL CYCLE

▶ **The first day of the menstrual cycle. The thickened lining of the uterus is shed, along with some blood. This is called a period.**

At the same time, an egg cell starts to mature in the ovary because of a message from the FSH hormone from the pituitary gland. The egg cell grows in a tiny sac called a follicle.

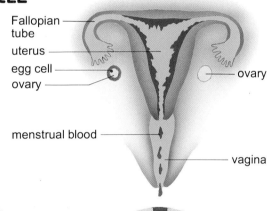

Fallopian tube

uterus

egg cell

ovary

ovary

menstrual blood

vagina

28 days

▼ **By about day 7 estrogen is being produced by the follicle, and this makes a new lining grow in the uterus.**

egg cell being matured

lining of uterus

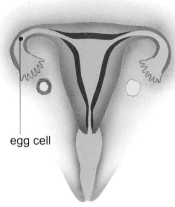

egg cell

▲ **If the egg is not fertilized by a sperm, the lining in the uterus will not be needed. It begins to break away. In a few days the next period will start.**

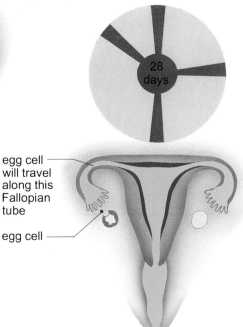

egg cell will travel along this Fallopian tube

egg cell

◀ **The pituitary gland produces LH which makes the mature egg, or ovum, burst out of the follicle. This is called ovulation.**

The empty follicle starts to produce a hormone called progesterone, which makes the lining of the uterus grow soft for a fertilized egg to nestle in and grow.

PERSONAL MATTERS

The parts of your body that are for producing babies are mostly inside. Once they begin working, during puberty, you will see signs outside. Girls begin to have periods about once a month. Boys will produce semen. Part of growing up is learning how to deal with these changes responsibly.

I'm not well

A MAJOR EVENT

I can't go swimming today

It's my visitor

I've got the curse

Can't wash my hair this week

These girls all have one thing in common. They have a slight blood loss from the vagina known as a period. From their comments, and the stories you might have heard, you will know that some people have very strange ideas about periods. However, a period is simply the visible part of the menstrual cycle, when the body sheds the thickened lining of the uterus, along with some blood.

A NEAT SOLUTION

The amount of blood lost is not usually very much, but girls and women do need to wear something to absorb it. Today there is a choice of pads, some of which have a sticky strip to hold them inside ordinary underwear. The pads need to be changed every few hours, and the soiled ones disposed of. Some girls prefer using tampons. These are small cylinders of absorbent material that slip inside the vagina. A range of sizes is available. They have a string attached so they can easily be pulled out. They *can't* get lost inside. It is very important to change a tampon every few hours. Otherwise, infections can develop. Tampons are easy to flush away.

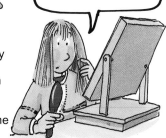

Q Pads or tampons—what should I use?

A Pads are probably easier to use when you first begin learning how to deal with periods. The small size should be enough to start with, and they won't make strange bulges through your clothes.

Tampons, which slip inside the vagina, are a good idea once you are used to periods. They offer even greater freedom: you can even go swimming if you use tampons.

Q Why don't I have a period regularly every month?

A When the pituitary gland and ovaries first begin to produce the hormones which control your period, they may not have settled down into a regular rhythm. The ovaries are still maturing and it can take time for them to work fully in producing their hormones and mature egg cells. All this means that it may be several months before you start to have periods regularly.

Q I was expecting my period just before my exams, but it didn't come. What's wrong?

A Sometimes when you are worried about something—exams, for instance, or a big change in your life—periods can be late. They may even stop for a few months. When everything settles the periods will return to normal.

Q My sister says periods are awful. Will mine be like that?

A Some people feel uncomfortable on the first day of a period. Think how your hand would feel if you had scraped it: it would ache a bit. The uterus can ache too. It sounds as if your sister is one of those people who have quite a lot of pain. Simple pain killers could help her for the first few hours. However, you are different. You might have little or no pain.

Q My mom is really awful just before her period and yells at me. Are the two things connected?

A Yes. One hormone, progesterone, which is produced after the egg is shed affects a number of things. It makes the body retain more water and it makes the breasts swell. At this time, women can feel uncomfortable. The hormone also affects the emotions, and makes some people irritable. This phase is called pre-menstrual syndrome, or PMS. It doesn't often happen to young people, and it doesn't happen to everyone.

Q I'm worried that I'll start my periods one day at school and won't have any sanitary protection.

A It isn't easy to tell when your first period is going to start. You might notice that your breasts become a bit enlarged—but you might not. Don't worry, though. The blood loss isn't heavy at first. You'll probably notice a slight staining in your underwear when you go to the toilet. If you don't have any pads, ask a female teacher. Schools usually keep some supplies on hand.

When you know you're likely to have periods, you can carry a tampon or pad with you—"just in case". They often come ready wrapped, and are small enough to hide in your school bag or purse.

AWKWARD MOMENTS

Once puberty starts, a boy may find that his penis gets stiff all by itself. He may find he can make this happen by thinking about girls.

Sometimes semen squirts out of the penis. This is called an ejaculation. When it happens during dreams, a boy will wake up with a wet, sticky patch on his pyjamas. These dreams are called wet dreams. The body is simply adjusting to becoming adult.

Once puberty has started, the penis also secretes smegma, which is whitish and thick. This collects under the foreskin of uncircumcised boys, and it needs to be washed away.

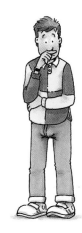

Q My girl cousin, who is about the same age as me, came to visit last weekend. When I saw her, my penis sort of stood up. What should I do?

A Every sympathy! That can be a bit embarrassing. I bet you don't even like your cousin as a girlfriend. It's just the way your body is. There isn't anything you can do, except try thinking about something else.

Q I've read that I should wash under the foreskin, but it won't roll back. Does this matter?

A This is a problem for a few boys. If the foreskin is too tight to be rolled back, you might get infections developing underneath. You should see a doctor, who will decide if you need to have the foreskin removed. The operation is called circumcision. It is done under general anesthetic.

Q Why do some boys have smaller penises than other boys?

A People are all different, and it is a simple fact that some boys do have smaller penises than others. The main disadvantage is that they can suffer some cruel teasing while they are growing up. However, size makes no difference to how well the penis "works".

SHAPING UP

Once you reach puberty, you change from looking like a child to looking more like a grown-up. If you begin to look grown-up before most of your friends, you may feel a bit strange. Just look at grown-up people around you! All shapes and sizes of them can look really good. So can you!

A WOMANLY SHAPE

During puberty girls begin to develop a curvy shape. When a girl's ovaries begin to produce estrogen, this hormone carries messages causing her breasts to begin to grow. At first, they are just little swellings behind the nipples. As each month goes by the breasts become larger and more rounded. The breasts are designed to produce milk when a woman has a baby and, from the time of puberty, the glands inside grow in readiness.

The hips also change. If you put your hands on either side of your waist and press down you will feel a bone. This bone is part of the pelvis, which forms a circular shape. The pelvis grows in a certain way depending on the message sent by the hormones. In girls, the hormones make the pelvis grow wider, so that there is plenty of room for a baby to pass through at birth.

A MANLY SHAPE

Boys develop differently. Their hormones make the pelvis stay longer and narrower, their shoulders grow wider and their muscles larger. Boys do not develop breasts. A few boys find that the area around their nipples does seem to swell. Even when this happens, it is hardly noticeable, and the swelling soon goes away once the hormones have sorted themselves out.

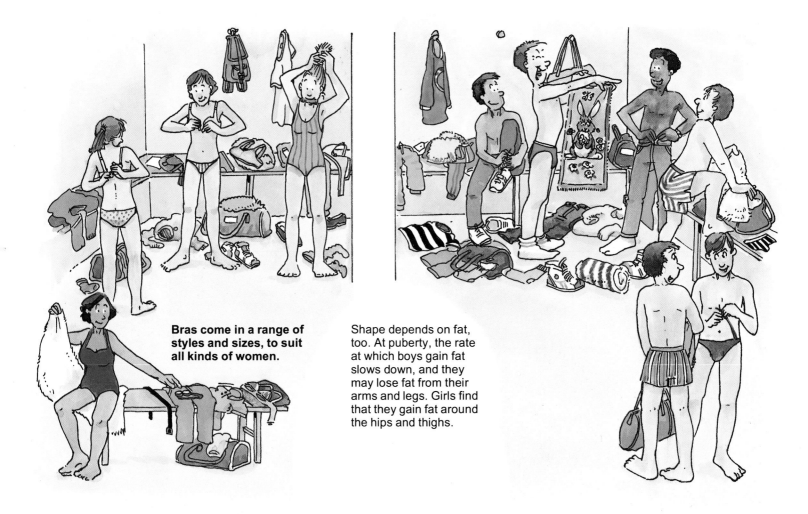

Bras come in a range of styles and sizes, to suit all kinds of women.

Shape depends on fat, too. At puberty, the rate at which boys gain fat slows down, and they may lose fat from their arms and legs. Girls find that they gain fat around the hips and thighs.

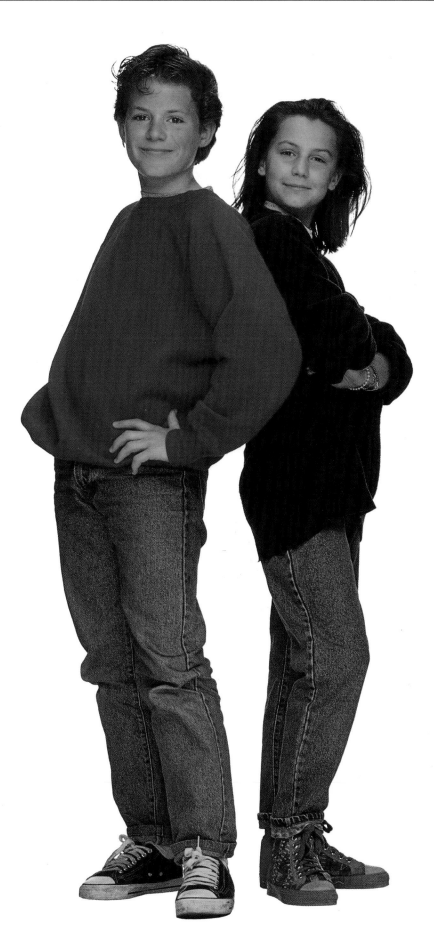

WEIGHTY MATTERS

Fashion magazines show all kinds of glamorous pictures of people with shapely bodies, all looking wonderful in the latest clothes. The good news is that as you develop a grown-up shape you'll be able to choose grown-up clothes. The problem is that some people begin to worry that they don't look like the fashion models.

Your actual shape depends on the special pattern written in each cell of your body and which you have inherited from your parents. You won't look exactly like either of them, but you will have some kind of family likeness. You can't change the way your bones grow!

In most cases, you can change how fat or thin you are. It depends on what you eat. If you want to look as good as possible, you need to be the right weight for your height. Too fat or too thin and you won't feel as good.

ANOREXIA

Some people worry that dieting may lead to a condition know as anorexia nervosa. This is a serious condition, in which some people are so concerned about not eating that they may slowly starve themselves to death. They see themselves as fat even though they are desperately thin. People who have it need special help. However, ordinary dieting doesn't cause anorexia.

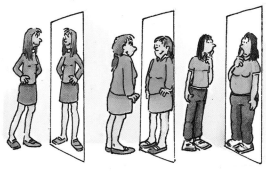

People are normally realistic about whether they are fat or thin. Someone who is anorexic has a mistaken view of their body shape.

As you grow up you will notice changes to your skin. It will begin to grow hair in some places. It may break out in pimples on your face.

A HAIRY TIME

During puberty, hair begins to grow on different parts of your body. Male hormones, called androgens, make it grow. Boys produce androgens in the testes, but both boys and girls make some in glands that are found on top of the kidneys. These are the adrenal glands.

Girls will grow hair in the pubic area called the mons. It may also grow over the large lips at the entrance to the vagina. Girls will grow some underarm hair too.

Boys are generally more hairy than girls, because they produce higher levels of the androgens which make the hair grow. The hair in the pubic area usually grows higher up the abdomen. More hair may grow on the chest, arms and legs. Boys also grow hair on their faces. Unless they want a mustache and beard, they have to shave this off.

SMOOTH TALKING

How much hair do you want on your body? In some countries people think that dark body hair is very beautiful. In others, they go to all lengths to get rid of it. Beards and mustaches are sometimes in fashion, sometimes not.

Shaving is probably the easiest and cheapest way to get rid of unwanted hair. From the time they are about 14, most boys will have to shave once or twice a week at least if they do not want to grow a beard and mustache. An electric shaver is easy to use.

Girls may want to remove hair from their legs and their underarms, and shaving is one way of doing so. It is easy and cheap.

There are also waxes and creams which get rid of body hair. They are quite safe if you follow the instructions carefully.

In some countries girls are particularly embarrassed if they have facial hair, such as a fine, dark mustache. Special creams are available that bleach the hair to make it less noticeable.

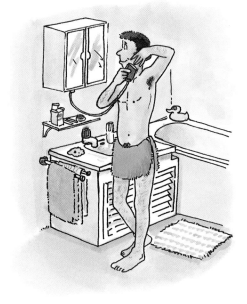

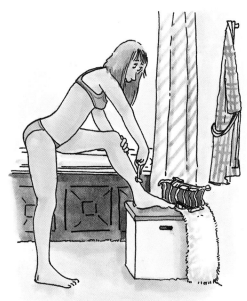

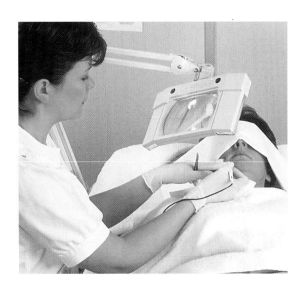

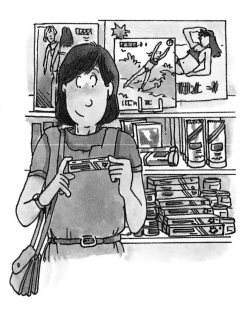

Electrolysis is the only permanent way of getting rid of body hair. It is best done by a professional beautician in a salon, who will use properly sterilized equipment. It is very expensive.

SKIN DEEP

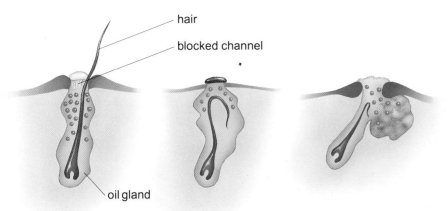

hair
blocked channel
oil gland

Skin is covered with tiny hairs, and each has a little oil gland (called a sebaceous gland) with it. Androgens—the hormones which make body hair grow—make these glands work overtime. At the same time, the tiny channel from the oil gland to the surface thickens, and so the oil may get blocked in. If it is completely blocked, it produces a pimple called a white-head.

If the channel remains open and some oil reaches the surface it turns black. This is because it mixes with oxygen, not because a person hasn't washed properly.

If the block makes the oil burst the channel and leak out sideways below the skin, it causes a large red spot. This is acne.

Almost all boys and girls are affected to some extent by acne. The problem usually goes away at about age 18 or 19.

FACING REALITY

Some people get so embarrassed about their skin that they hide. Don't miss out on the fun of growing up. There are some dos and don'ts that can help to keep acne under control.

● DO enjoy your food. Acne is not caused by diet.

● DO cleanse your skin carefully. Washing with soap can make pimples worse. You can buy special washing lotions for acne.

● DON'T pick or squeeze. Most pimples won't leave permanent marks on your skin, but if you pick them they will leave a scar.

● DON'T wear your hair over your face. It might hide the pimples, but it makes them worse.

● DON'T suffer silently. Lots can be done to get rid of acne. If you have really bad pimples, your doctor will be able to suggest special treatment.

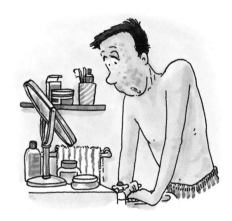

THE VOICE OF MATURITY

Little girls and little boys have similar voices, but grown-up men and women have very different voices because their vocal cords develop differently. The voice box, or larynx, is in the throat. Inside there are vocal cords, and as air passes through they vibrate to make sound waves. If you put your finger on the front of your throat you will be able to feel a lump. This is the larynx.

The larynx of a newborn boy or girl is very tiny and the cords are only about $1/10$ inch long. As the larynx get bigger and the cords longer, the high-pitched cry of the baby gives way to the deeper tone of the child. Just before puberty both boys and girls will have vocal cords that are about $11/16$ inch long.

Now comes the change. During puberty a girl's vocal cords grow to about $7/8$ inch, but a boy's grow to more than $11/8$ inch. In a boy, the tiny muscles controlling the cords have difficulty doing so while they are growing so rapidly. Sometimes they do not hold them at the right tension. The voice may wobble, like a stringed instrument being tuned as the string is tightened or loosened. The boy's voice is usually said to be "breaking". After a while, the muscles relearn their duties!

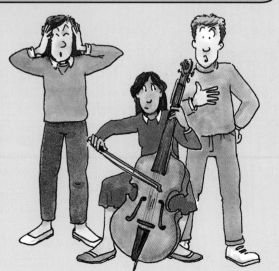

YOUR OWN PERSON

One of the best things about growing up is finding out who you really are. At this time of your life, everything seems to be changing—not only your appearance, but also your likes and dislikes. You start developing your own opinions: what you think is important, what you believe in, what you value.

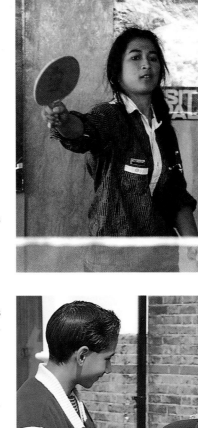

UPS AND DOWNS

Most of the time there are reasons for the way you feel. You feel good because things are going well. You feel worried because something needs sorting out. It's important to take notice of your feelings. They help you avoid trouble and solve problems.

During puberty the dramatic changes going on in your body also affect the way you feel. You will notice that sometimes you feel happy, and confident that everything in your life is going fine. Then the smallest thing can suddenly make you feel that the world is terrible, that nothing will ever work out and that no one understands.

Mood swings like this are very common. They are simply caused by surges of hormones. Think about what it's like to be on a playground swing. The world sometimes seems near and sometimes far away. It's not the world that's moving—it's you on the swing. Even when your mood changes and you feel that everything is going really badly, remember that it could well be you who has changed position. Your life is not suddenly worse than it was before; things are not really as bad as they seem.

WHAT'S IT ALL ABOUT?

Just as the parts of your body all have functions, so your whole body has a function. The God who made us did not leave us to live life as best we can. He provided guidelines for living, which can be found in the Bible. If people are to be happy, they need to live as they were designed to do: caring for each other and looking after the world and all the creatures in it. So, even when you feel down, you can know that God thinks you are very important. You have a part to play in the world!

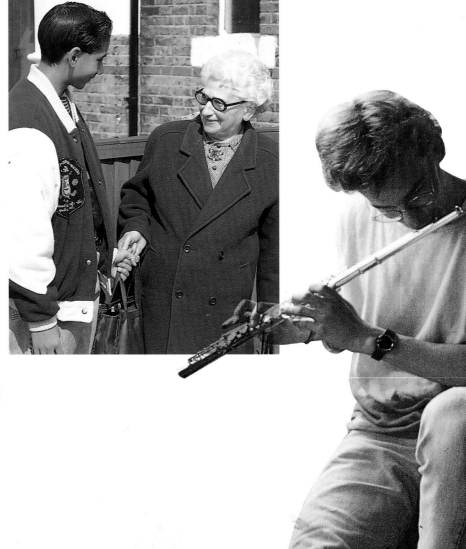

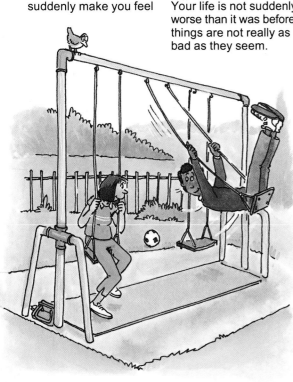

THE REAL YOU

What are you really like? Do you enjoy camping, or is it your family who are wild about it? Do you hate music, or is it that you don't really get on with the music teacher in your school right now? Is anything you do any good?

You will find you are good at some things, and interested in them. Other things will bore you, or you will find them more of a challenge. At times you will probably wish you were more like someone else—someone smarter/better looking/more talented/more popular.

You are a special person, with a special contribution to make in the world. Learn to recognize your own talents, and be glad.

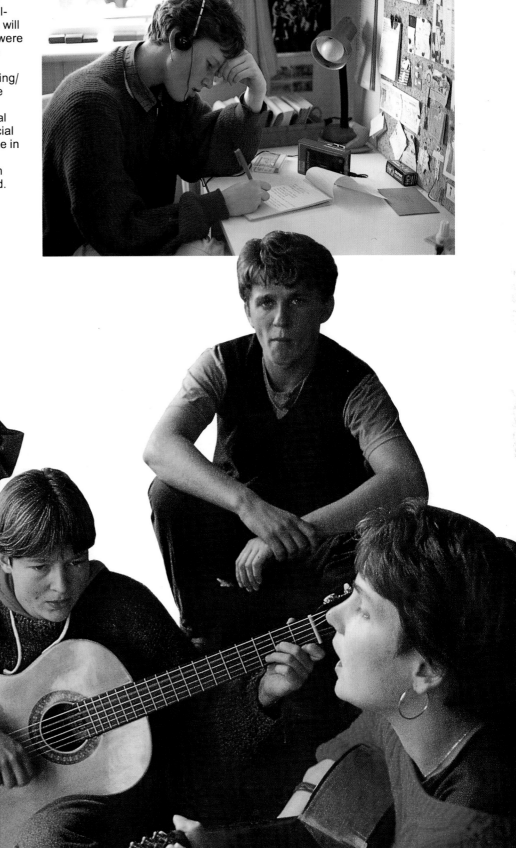

'Families are great. They look after you, buy you nice things, give you lots of laughs.'

'Families are terrible. Parents nag. They treat you like a kid. They won't let you do anything on your own. Brothers and sisters borrow your things without asking.'

Families can be all of these things. However, when God made people, he designed them to live in families. Young children need grown-ups to care for them and guide them until they are older and can be responsible for themselves. Right now, you're beginning to grow up. How far can you manage by yourself?

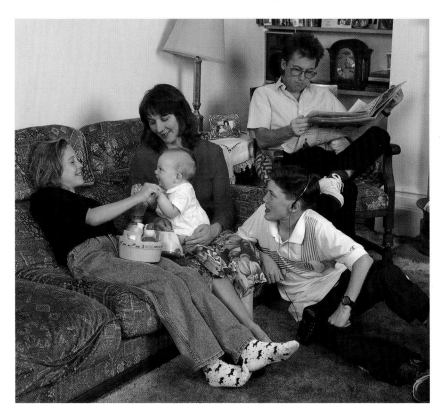

TEACHING THE GROWN-UPS

Won't they ever learn that you're not a child? Grown-ups can be very frustrating! *Be home on time. Tell us where you're going—and who you're going with—and what you plan to do. Do your homework. Turn the music down. Turn the television off. Leave your shoes here. Put the dirty laundry there.*

However, imagine how they see things.

The adults in your family remember you from the time you were tiny. If you've met anyone when *they* were a baby, you'll know how easy it is to think of them as still being a baby! People need time to see just how grown up you really are. It helps if you show how grown-up you have become by what you do.

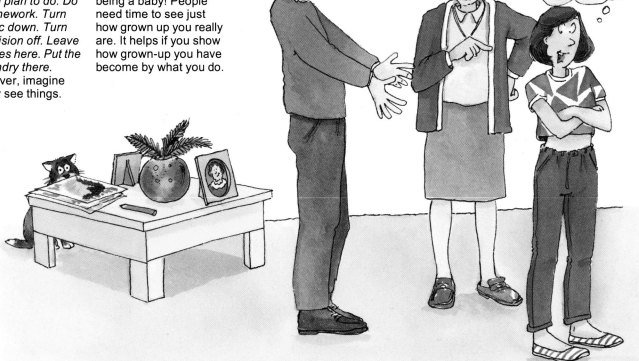

SOUND ADVICE

Have you ever thought that families could use some guidelines? The Bible has some interesting ones. God advises parents not be so unreasonable that they drive their kids insane! Quite right, too. He advises children to respect their parents. After all, they have done quite a lot for you. Listen to what they have to say, and try to find things that you can agree on.

ALL BY YOURSELF

Doing things all by yourself is not easy. It's nice to go out by yourself—but it can be handy to have someone come to take you home, particularly after dark. It's fun choosing your own clothes, but even more so if someone else is paying. Your room is strictly private and no one should come in even to pick up your stuff, but it's important to have clean clothes ready when you have an invitation to a special party.

Of course you want to learn how to do things by yourself, and it's important that you do learn! However, you know that you like someone to help out at times. Don't be too hard on your family if they rush in to help at a time when you don't feel you need it.

THINK FOR YOURSELF

Here are some easy things to do to show that you know how to think for yourself.

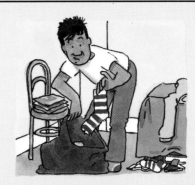

Take charge of your own belongings and your living space.

Sort out mistakes. As you begin to make your own choices you are likely to make a few bad ones. Never mind, you'll know better next time.

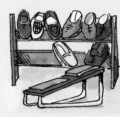

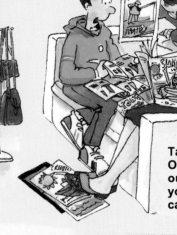

Don't just follow the crowd. Think about what you want to do, what you think is right and wrong.

Talk things through. Often, you can work out a way in which you and your family can agree.

Dare to say you're sorry. You know that you'd want others to apologize to you.

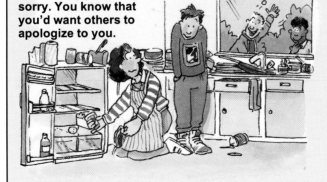

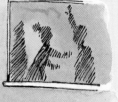

Be glad that people care about you. Sometimes you may wish that your family lived on another planet. Other times, you'll be glad they are around to help.

Hooray for friends. They make you feel wanted, they care about you, and they don't boss you around. You like them, and you want to spend time with them. You have the same likes and dislikes.

Oddly, the grown-ups in your family do not like all your friends. They complain about you spending too much time with friends when you should be at home. They claim that you let your friends decide what you do, where you go, the type of music you listen to, and even the clothes you wear.

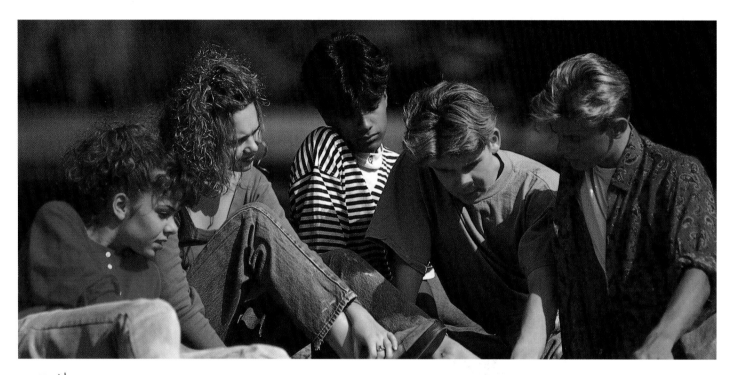

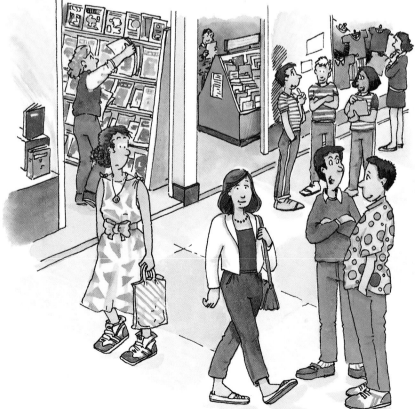

FOLLOWING THE CROWD

You want to have your own style. Now is the time to start developing it. The clothes you wear, the magazines you read, the music you listen to—you want these things to reflect the real you.

It would be nice to know that people were looking at you and thinking: What a great choice! It's hard to know sometimes what makes a good choice.

When you first start choosing things for yourself, such as music and clothes, you may choose things that people tell you are good, without really thinking whether or not you agree. You might not go along with what the grown-ups in your family think, but you will probably trust your friends. Or what the popular magazines say. Or what the advertisements in the magazines claim.

Of course you don't want to be too different from other people you mix with. You want to fit in. However, you can discover from your successes and your mistakes what really does appeal to you.

WHOSE STANDARDS?

You're not only making choices about what to buy. You are also having to choose a lifestyle that suits you. Lots of young people experiment with different lifestyles, and this can drive the people who care for them frantic with worry. There are good reasons why: some experiments can cause real damage.

- **Cigarettes.** All bad news here: smoking is expensive and leaves a smell of stale tobacco hanging around you. Worse, the poisons in cigarettes cause cancer and other diseases of the arteries and lungs. Once you start smoking, it's hard to give up. The most sensible choice is not to start.

- **Drugs.** Some people try drugs to find out what effect they have. It's worth finding out some other way. At the time, drugs may make a person feel that life is wonderful. Then again,

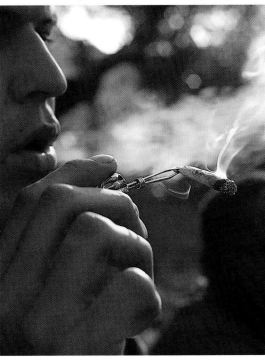

they may make a person feel that life is so awful they'd be better off dead. Drugs are very habit-forming, and over time they can damage your body. Many drug addicts do die young.

Never puff a cigarette that someone wants to pass around. If you are offered any strange fluid or powder to sniff, taste or inject, say no.

- **Alcohol.** Alcohol isn't as addictive as other drugs, and many people enjoy an occasional drink with a meal with no bad effects. Nevertheless, it is a drug, and it slows the body down and makes a person feel relaxed and sleepy. Even a small amount can slow a person down so much that they can't drive safely. Too much at one time can make a person lose control of themselves. The next day, they feel embarrassed— and ill. Too much alcohol over a long period can permanently damage your body.

Q There's a gang of kids at my school who are always teasing me, saying I've got an ugly nose and stuff like that. They make me feel miserable. What can I do?

A They sound like a mean group. You have a real challenge here. First, take a look at yourself. They succeed in making you miserable because, deep down, you are a bit worried about your looks. But that's the way you were made, and you look

fine. Think of all the people who aren't sneering at you. So next time this gang comes by simply look at them and say, or even just think, no, I'm fine. They'll know they aren't getting through, and they'll leave you alone.

Of course, while your confidence grows, you could simply avoid them as much as possible.

Q Everyone else in my class seems to have friends. I

don't seem to have any. What's wrong with me? At break, I just hang around with the little kids for something to do.

A Nothing is wrong with you. It's just that other people in your class seem a bit busy with each other right now. They probably think you're having fun with the little kids. Maybe you are. If you want to make friends with people in your class, perhaps you'll have to ask if you can join in with them. A few

might turn you away, but there are bound to be some who are glad to think that YOU like THEM.

Q I told my best friend something really private—to do with my family—and now he's let it slip to other people. I feel totally let down. What can I do?

A Even the best of friends can let you down. It could be that your

friend really was being unkind, but it's more likely that he told other people without thinking. Remind him that it is a topic that you wanted to keep private. Then forgive him this mistake and get on with being friends.

LOVE IS...

There are different kinds of love. Love for family, love for friends, love for our pets, and even love for places and things. From the time you start growing up, the love that comes to mind most often is the type that makes your heart beat faster!

GOING OUT TOGETHER

It all starts with interest in the opposite sex: girls stop thinking that boys are horrible, and boys stop thinking that girls are weird. The idea of having a special boyfriend or girlfriend becomes appealing.

The sex hormones make this change happen. As well as making the body develop, they change the way boys and girls think about each other. It is quite normal to have romantic dreams about a special relationship. You may admire someone from afar—a rock star, perhaps, or a teacher—and spend ages thinking about being with them.

At this stage, the easiest way to get to know people of the opposite sex is to meet in a group, where you can still have your old friends around. It is hard to know just what to say and do, so being with others helps.

Gradually the group will start to pair off. Boys and girls will go out together and get to know each other better.

Of course, you may discover that the person you get to know isn't really the kind of person you relate to easily. You—or the other person—may decide to end the special friendship. And that can be a very difficult time. However, you shouldn't feel guilty about suggesting that

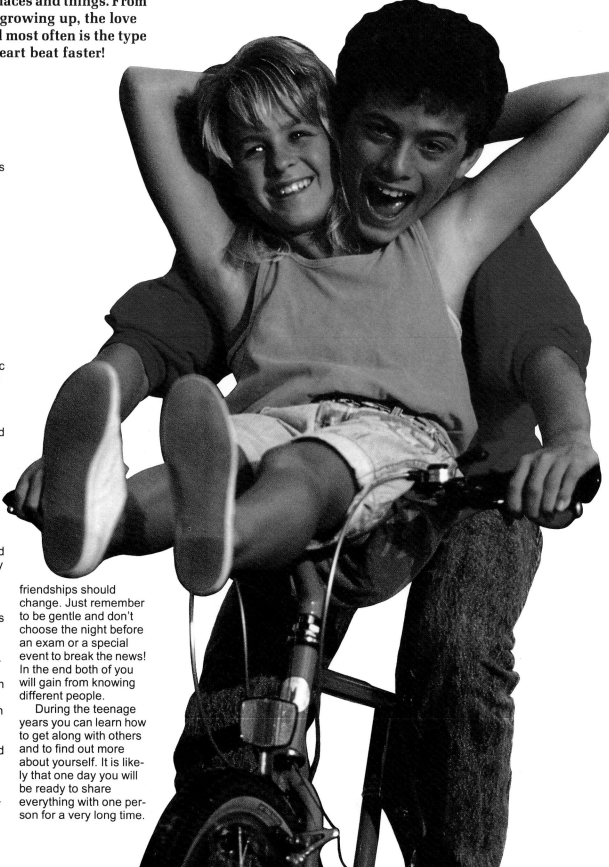

friendships should change. Just remember to be gentle and don't choose the night before an exam or a special event to break the news! In the end both of you will gain from knowing different people.

During the teenage years you can learn how to get along with others and to find out more about yourself. It is likely that one day you will be ready to share everything with one person for a very long time.

PARTY SURVIVAL GUIDE

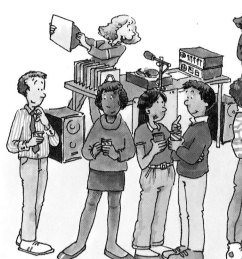

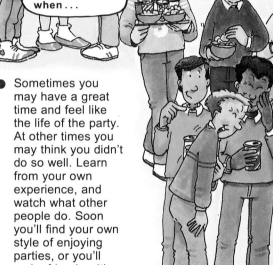

So after I'd been shopping, I went back home, washed my hair, dried my hair, ate my supper...

Did you see the bit in the game when...

A party invitation, and what do you LOOK like? Is your hair right? Are your nails clean? Then there's your face: what about the PIMPLES? What are you going to wear? Why do you look so fat/thin/flat/bulgy?

Eventually your family will hammer so hard on the bathroom door that you have to get out and go to the party. You've done your best: now there are other things to think about.

● Do you have interesting things to talk about? Who will you talk to first?

● Will you listen to others talking? Who do you like to listen to?

● Will you join in the party, or do you prefer helping with the food or the music?

● What will you do if SOMEONE SPECIAL is there? What will you do if that person is not there?

● Sometimes you may have a great time and feel like the life of the party. At other times you may think you didn't do so well. Learn from your own experience, and watch what other people do. Soon you'll find your own style of enjoying parties, or you'll make friends with the kinds of people who hate parties!

LOVING RELATIONSHIPS

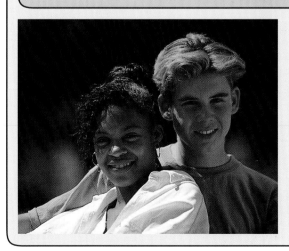

How would you answer the question, "What is love?" Here is one description of what love is:

"Love is patient, love is kind. It does not envy, it does not boast, it is not proud. It is not rude, it is not self-seeking, it is not easily angered, it keeps no record of wrongs... It always protects, always trusts, always hopes, always perseveres.

Love never fails."

The apostle Paul wrote that description in a letter to people in Corinth (Greece) nearly 2000 years ago. He was telling them about the kind of love God wanted them to have for each other: the kind of love everyone could see in the life of Jesus Christ. It is about really caring for another person, wanting the best for them,

whatever happens.

You can read the rest of Paul's letter in the New Testament in the Bible, in the book called I Corinthians. It applies to all our relationships, not just those between a boy and a girl, or a man and a woman.

PARTNERS

What is the purpose of all the changes of growing up? Your body gets ready for one part of the process of making babies. Your feelings make you interested in members of the opposite sex, who have the other part of the equipment. God's plan is that a man and a woman should get together to form a loving relationship that will be the basis of a new family.

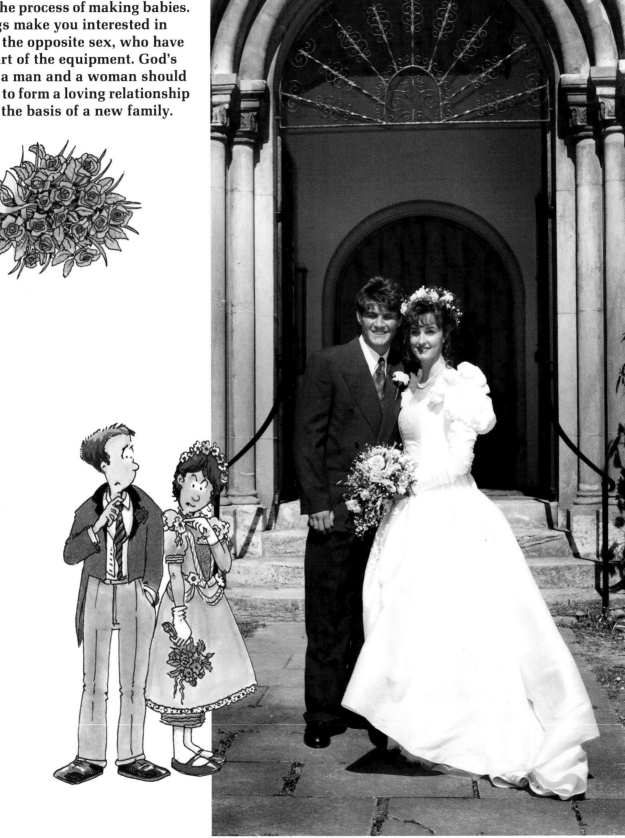

FRIENDS FOREVER

When a man and a woman decide that they really enjoy being together, they may decide to get married. This means that they make a special promise to stay together for the rest of their lives. In that time they may be rich and successful or they may be short of money. They may have the strength and energy to do lots of exciting things, or one or both may be ill and need a lot of special care. No matter. They will look after each other and care for each other. There has to be a lot of talking about the kind of future they would like to have together before they make this promise.

They also promise to share their bodies with each other in a special way: they will have sexual intercourse, which will bring them a lot of pleasure in itself and will very likely lead to babies!

A PERFECT MATCH

The book of Genesis in the Bible tells us that when God made people, he made male and female—man and woman. It explains that they were designed so that they could help each other. A man and a woman are the perfect match for each other.

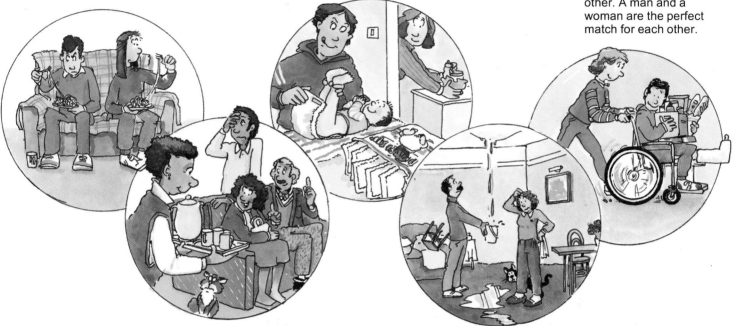

MAKING LOVE

Sexual intercourse is called making love, because it is the sign of a very special, loving relationship. Intercourse starts when the penis is placed inside the vagina and is completed when the penis is removed, but there is a lot more to it than that!

Sexual feelings build up gradually as the couple kiss and caress. Once intercourse has begun the penis is moved up and down inside the vagina until the most exciting stage is reached. This peak of excitement is

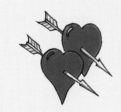

called orgasm. In the man, it triggers the release of semen into the vagina. The woman can also have an orgasm as the clitoris is stimulated. It often takes longer for her to reach this stage, and a lot depends on the skill and gentleness of her partner.

Making love can be a deeply satisfying way to express love and togetherness. It is part of God's plan to have babies born to a couple who can provide them with a loving home in which to grow up.

SEX BEFORE MARRIAGE

It is against the law for children to have sex. This law is to protect young people from having sex before they can fully understand the consequences of what they are doing. The age at which they are allowed to decide is called the age of consent. In many countries this is 16.

Even after that age, sex outside of marriage is against the instructions given to us by the God who made us. Sexual intercourse is meant to be the most loving part of a marriage, in which partners try to give pleasure as well as to receive it. This sharing of their bodies is a delight in itself and something that helps to make their relationship even more close and loving. Outside a loving marriage, sex becomes a rather selfish way to get a few thrills. Worse, it often results in feelings of guilt, tears and possibly worry about an unwanted pregnancy or infections that are transmitted sexually. Often there is disappointment with the act itself, because it has been rushed and uncomfortable. If the relationship ends, the people involved feel more deeply hurt than if they had been less intimate.

A NEW LIFE BEGINS

Sexual intercourse is needed for humans to make babies. A baby begins with just two cells—one from the man and one from the woman. As a result, the child inherits some of the looks and characteristics of both its parents.

AN INCREDIBLE JOURNEY

An enormous number of sperms are deposited in the vagina during intercourse. Only the strongest survive the journey to the Fallopian tube, where the egg cell can be fertilized. Many sperms try to break down the wall of the egg cell, but only one actually breaks through.

This sperm then unites with the egg. This is fertilization.

Soon after fertilization the new cell splits into two, then four. Eventually a clump of cells forms, looking rather like a miniature blackberry.

The clump of cells changes from a solid mass to a tiny balloon filled with fluid. Special cells grow on the outside which will help it to burrow into the lining of the uterus. Timing is important. If the little clump of cells arrives too soon, it will be unable to settle in the lining of the uterus and will die.

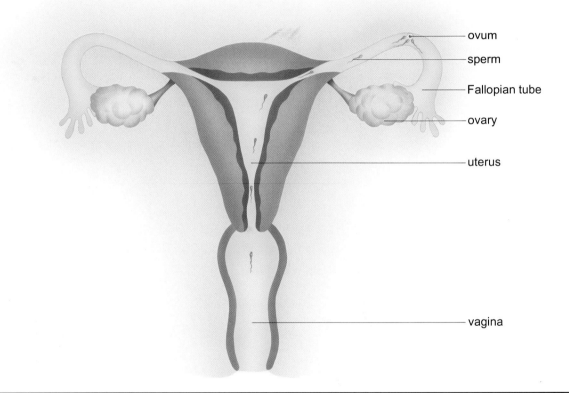

- ovum
- sperm
- Fallopian tube
- ovary
- uterus
- vagina

PROGRAMMED FOR LIFE

From the time the successful sperm penetrates the egg and fertilization takes place, all the information needed to make a new person is contained in that one cell. It contains 46 tiny chromosomes—23 from the sperm and 23 from the egg. If you were able to look at the chromosomes through a powerful microscope you would see that they are like tiny threads, arranged in pairs. Each thread is made up of hundreds of sections which are called genes. It is the genes that will decide the color of the baby's hair, its height—in fact everything about the way its body grows.

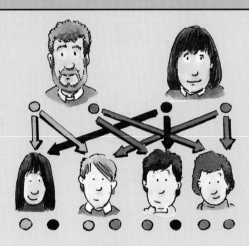

Everyone has two genes which give instructions for their hair color—one from their mother and one from their father. The gene for dark hair is the strongest and overrules the genes for other hair colors. The gene for red hair is the weakest and a person will only have red hair if they receive red hair genes from both parents.

2 x 2 = 4

Body cells increase in number by dividing: one cell becomes two, two become four, and so on. In fact, by the time a baby is born, the single fertilized egg cell will have increased to 200 thousand million cells. Every time a cell divides, the chromosomes are copied and then split in half so that the new cell has exactly the same chromosomes and genes.

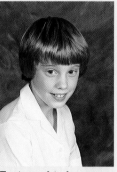
chromosomes of egg

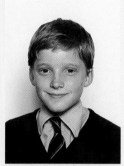
chromosomes of sperm

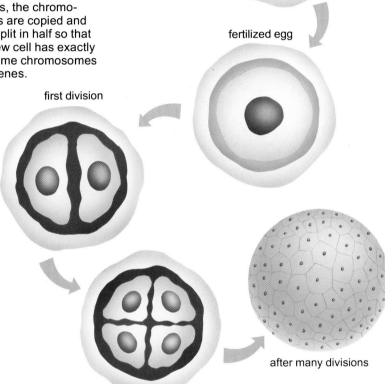
fertilized egg

first division

second division

after many divisions

BOY OR GIRL?

Two of the 46 chromosomes are known as the "sex" chromosomes because they carry a special code that will determine whether the new baby will be a boy or a girl. Girls have an XX code and boys have an XY code. Eggs always carry an X chromosome, but sperms will have either an X or Y code, so the sperm is responsible for producing a boy or a girl.

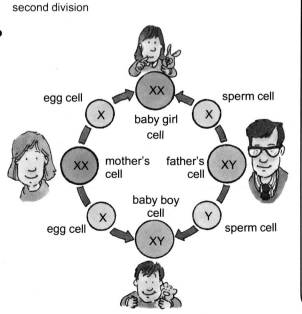

egg cell — X
XX baby girl cell
sperm cell — X
mother's cell — XX
father's cell — XY
baby boy cell
egg cell — X
XY
Y — sperm cell
XY

TWINS

Sometimes two egg cells leave the ovary at the same time. Since there are many sperms waiting for them to arrive in the Fallopian tube, they can both be fertilized. Two separate babies grow inside the uterus at the same time. The babies share the same birthday, but apart from that they are no more alike than any other brother and sister. These are called fraternal twins.

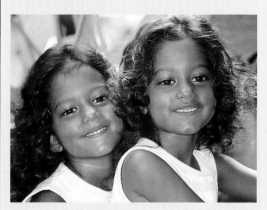

Fraternal twins are not necessarily of the same sex.

Sometimes, soon after fertilization the new growing cluster of cells splits in half to form two babies with exactly the same pattern of genes and chromosomes. They will grow into identical babies.

Identical twins are almost indistinguishable. They are always the same sex.

It takes about 38 weeks for a human being to develop from a fertilized cell to a fully grown baby. However, it is possible to see a picture of the developing baby. The pictures are created by a special technique called ultrasound. This technique bounces sounds too high to hear through the mother's skin and on to the baby. The echoes bounce back from the baby and these sounds are turned into dots on a television monitor to make a picture.

Ultrasound picture of a baby at 8 weeks.

I TICK

In its early stages, the growing life is called an embryo. It looks something like a fish with a head forming at one end and a tail at the other. Yet even now the special cells starting to form the heart are beating. A thick stalk from its middle will grow into a long cord that will be a lifeline during pregnancy. This cord goes from the baby to its life-support system, called the placenta. This placenta is attached to the wall of the uterus. It filters oxygen and nutrients from the mother's blood into the baby's blood.

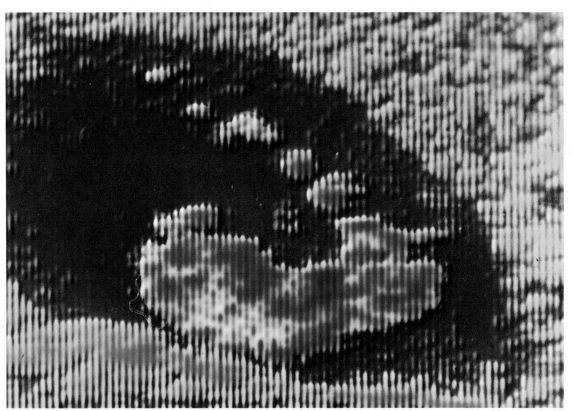

I WRIGGLE

By 12 weeks the growing life is a recognizable human being. Now it is called a fetus. You can see its head, body and arms quite clearly. The face has formed and the hands and feet have grown fingers and toes.

   The baby lies in a bag of fluid, called amniotic fluid, which protects it from bumps as its mother gets on with daily life.

Ultrasound picture of a baby at 12 weeks.

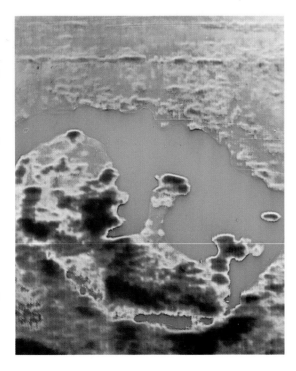

I KICK

The baby has been able to kick for a long time. By 18 weeks it is big enough and strong enough for the mother to feel the kicks. The first ones that can be noticed feel like a gentle fluttering. Later they will be a solid punch!

SLEEPING AND WAKING

By 28 weeks the baby clearly has times when it is awake and kicking, and other times when it is still and asleep. It continues to develop, getting ready for life in the open air.

I'M READY!

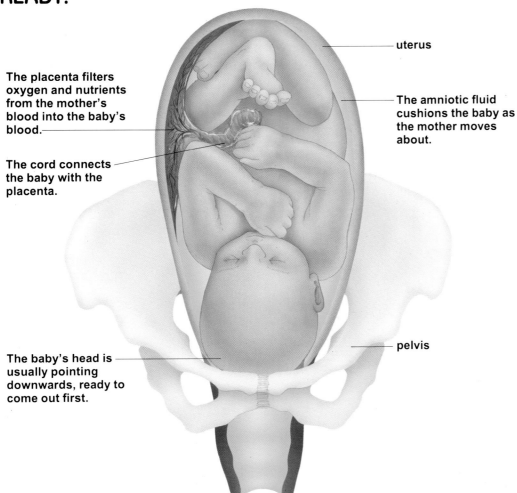

uterus

The placenta filters oxygen and nutrients from the mother's blood into the baby's blood.

The amniotic fluid cushions the baby as the mother moves about.

The cord connects the baby with the placenta.

pelvis

The baby's head is usually pointing downwards, ready to come out first.

CHECKING UP

During pregnancy a woman will have several check-ups to make sure that the baby is growing normally and that she is keeping well. A doctor can check on the progress of the baby by feeling it through the mother's body. Blood and urine tests and a blood pressure check also provide a way of making sure that everything is going well.

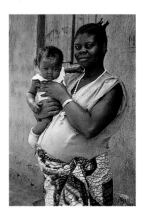

WHEN WILL BABY ARRIVE?

A pregnancy lasts about 38 weeks from the date the egg is fertilized, but it is hard to tell when fertilization takes place.

However, the egg cell is ready to be fertilized around the middle of a woman's monthly cycle. So, to calculate when a baby is due, a woman counts from the first day of her last menstrual period, which is about 2 weeks before fertilization. She counts those 2 weeks then adds 38 weeks, which makes 40 weeks.

A simple way to work out 40 weeks is to add 7 days and nine calendar months.

Can you work out the likely birth dates?

Last period began	Add 7 days	Add 9 months	
For example:			
3 Jan	10 Jan	=	10 Oct
18 Mar	25 Mar	=	?
26 Jul	2 Aug	=	?

MISCARRIAGE

A miscarriage is the ending of a pregnancy in the early weeks. It is also called a spontaneous abortion. A very large number of pregnancies—probably about 60 per cent—end even before the woman knows she is pregnant. The pregnancy will be expelled at the time of an expected period.

Many other pregnancies end naturally in the first three months. Usually the reason is that the pregnancy is not developing normally. A couple who has been looking forward to a baby will be very unhappy when this happens. They will mourn the loss of the baby that they were hoping for.

A fully developed baby is ready to survive in the world. Its body is fully working so that it can breathe air and digest its food. By this time, it has filled most of the space inside its mother's uterus. It is ready to come out.

The process of birth is called labor, because it is hard work. The mother's uterus has to work to push the baby out. The average length of labor for a woman having her first baby is about 12–18 hours, but it varies a lot. Labor has three stages.

WHAT DOES LABOR FEEL LIKE?

You know that your muscles can hurt if you do very hard work for a long time. The muscles that are used during labor are working very hard indeed, and this can cause pain. Women can take time before their baby is due to learn how to relax so that the pain doesn't frighten them. Instead, they can concentrate on letting their body work to deliver the baby. They can feel the head come out, and then the baby's body. There are also pain killers suitable for use during labor. The medical team assisting at the birth will administer them carefully.

STAGE 1

This is the longest part. It is the time when the lower part of the uterus opens to allow the baby to come out into the vagina. The muscles in the uterus work to push the baby down. They do this by contracting, which means they become hard and tense and get shorter. Labor always starts with contractions developing and getting stronger, but a woman may notice a discharge of fluid from the vagina first. Eventually, the contractions push the baby through the opening of the uterus, which is called the cervix.

At some stage, it is likely that the bag of fluid around the baby will break and the amniotic fluid will leak away.

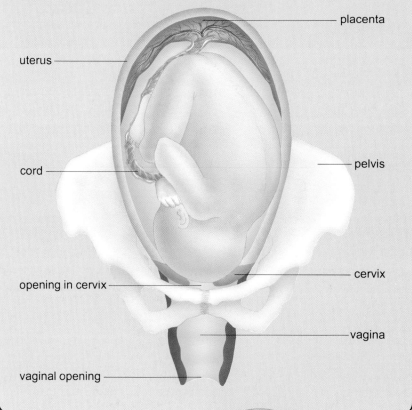

- placenta
- uterus
- cord
- opening in cervix
- vaginal opening
- pelvis
- cervix
- vagina

ANOTHER WAY OUT

Most babies lie in such a way inside the uterus that they come out head first. Some lie the other way around. When a baby comes out bottom first it is known as a breech birth.

In a few cases, the baby has difficulty being born through the vagina. Then doctors may decide to deliver the baby by an operation called a Caesarean section. The woman is given an anesthetic and a surgeon makes a cut through to the uterus and lifts the baby out. The cut is painful until it heals, as with any operation, and it leaves a small scar.

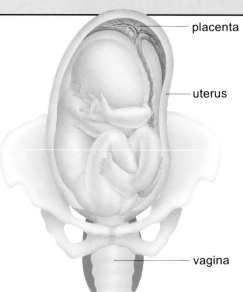

- placenta
- uterus
- vagina

STAGE 2

Once the cervix is open the second stage of labor begins. The uterus continues to push the baby down through the pelvis and out through the vagina. The mother will feel an urge to push too, and can in this way help to push her baby out. Once the head is out, the rest of the baby slips out easily. The cord that links the baby to its placenta is clamped or tied. It is then cut close to the baby's tummy to separate the baby from the placenta.

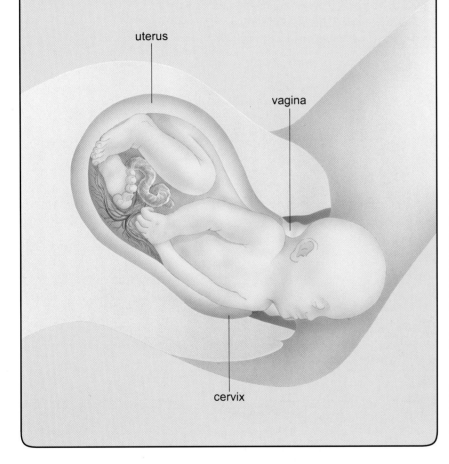

uterus

vagina

cervix

STAGE 3

After the baby is born, the placenta peels off the wall of the uterus. It leaves a large area that would normally bleed, but the uterus is suddenly much smaller, and as it contracts and tightens it clamps all the blood vessels shut.

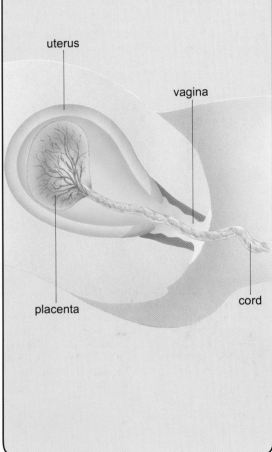

uterus

vagina

placenta

cord

WHAT ABOUT MEN?

The main work of delivering a baby has to be done by the mother! However, it is an experience that many couples want to share. The woman likes to have someone who can be helpful and comforting during labor, and the father is often the best person for the job. It is a real thrill for both mother and father to see the baby as soon as it is born.

From the birth day onwards the father can join in the work and the pleasure of looking after the baby.

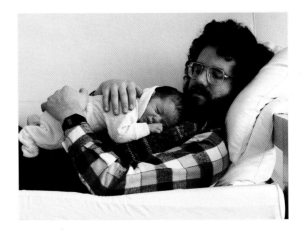

At birth the baby comes out of its own warm pool of water. It has to start breathing, taking in a first gulp of air and sometimes yelling as it does so! The baby is covered in a thick oil called vernix that has protected its skin from the water, and this can now be washed off.

A baby is not the same shape as a grown person. It has a large head for its size, and a tiny body. There is a soft spot on its head, covered only by a special, thick skin under the ordinary skin. This is so that the skull bones can overlap during labor, which means the head can be pushed out more easily. It will be a couple of years before the bones grow together. A little stump of cord will still be left on its tummy, and this will dry out and fall off in a few days, leaving a little dent, called the navel.

A baby may have masses of hair or none at all! It may be active or sleepy. Even though a newborn baby cannot do very much for itself, it is already a complete and very special person.

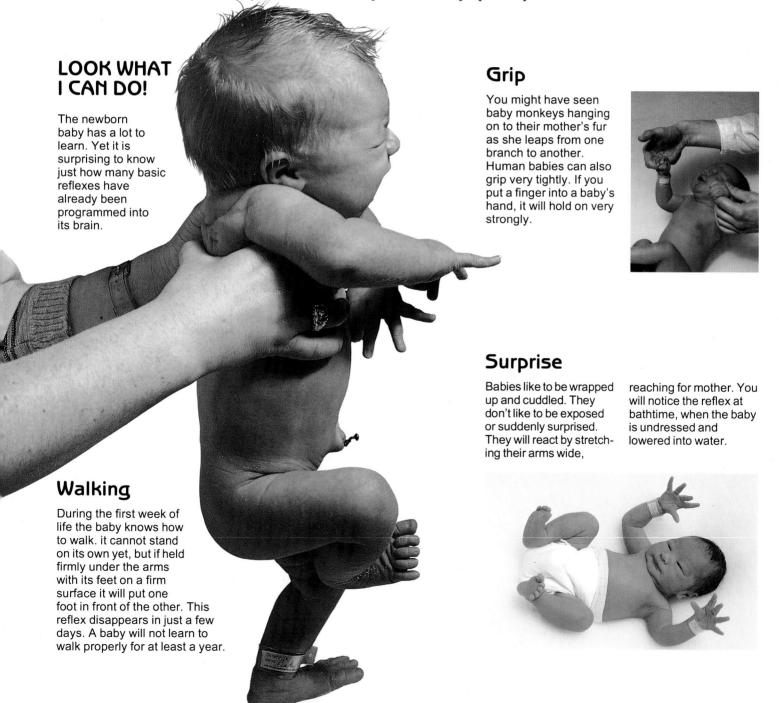

LOOK WHAT I CAN DO!

The newborn baby has a lot to learn. Yet it is surprising to know just how many basic reflexes have already been programmed into its brain.

Grip

You might have seen baby monkeys hanging on to their mother's fur as she leaps from one branch to another. Human babies can also grip very tightly. If you put a finger into a baby's hand, it will hold on very strongly.

Surprise

Babies like to be wrapped up and cuddled. They don't like to be exposed or suddenly surprised. They will react by stretching their arms wide, reaching for mother. You will notice the reflex at bathtime, when the baby is undressed and lowered into water.

Walking

During the first week of life the baby knows how to walk. it cannot stand on its own yet, but if held firmly under the arms with its feet on a firm surface it will put one foot in front of the other. This reflex disappears in just a few days. A baby will not learn to walk properly for at least a year.

WHAT DOES IT EAT?

Once the baby is born, the placenta in the mother's body is gone and its hormones disappear. This allows other hormones in her body to send messages to her breasts to make them produce milk. The baby sucks at the nipple to get the milk. It contains all the nutrients a baby needs for the first months of life.

It is also possible to buy substitutes for human milk that have been made from modified cows' milk. These can be useful if the mother is not around to feed her baby or has difficulty doing so. A baby's bottle has a teat with a tiny hole so that the baby can suck the milk.

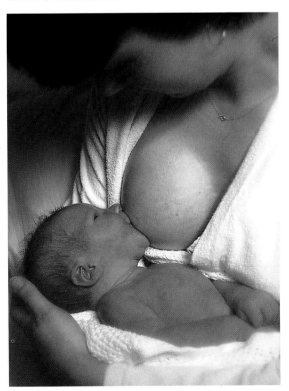

Feeding

When a baby feels something against its cheek it will hunt for it and suck. This reflex helps a baby suck milk from its mother's breast.

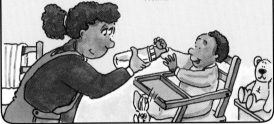

A FUNNY SMELL

Babies do not come toilet trained! They produce urine and feces when the body is ready to let them out. Today, most babies wear special garments to absorb the mess. These are changed when they are wet or dirty. The soiled garments may be of cloth, which needs to be washed, or paper, which can be disposed of.

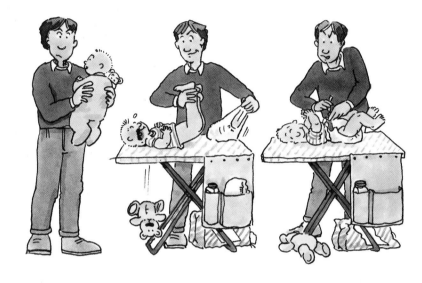

CRY BABY

Babies cannot talk. They will learn to do so in the first 3 years of life. In the meantime, they tell others when they need something by making crying noises. A crying baby needs something—perhaps milk, perhaps a cuddle.

Babies do not notice day and night while they are growing inside their mothers. For the first few weeks they need milk every couple of hours regardless of the time. When they are big enough they may sleep for several hours at a time, and eventually they learn to have this long sleep at night!

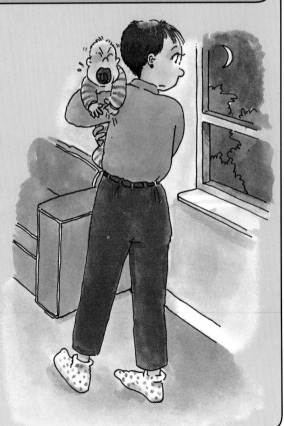

How many children make the best kind of family? None? One? Two or three? Ten? All over the world people have different views on how many children they want in the family.

Whatever a couple decides is the best size of family for them: it is good to plan, so that every child is wanted. Without some kind of planning, a couple could go on having children until the woman is no longer able to bear them, when she is approaching the age of 50. Depending on when a couple gets married, that could mean a great many children! Family planning helps them choose.

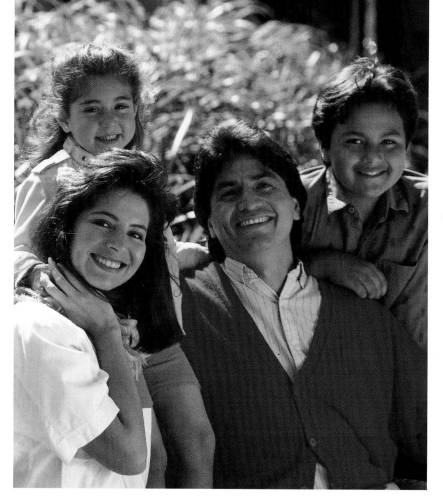

PLANNING FOR A BABY

Women release an egg cell each month, around the middle of a regular monthly cycle. Couples who want to have a baby should plan to have sexual intercourse at this time to increase their chances of having a baby.

On the other hand, couples who do not want to have a baby can plan to make love only at other times in the monthly cycle. This method reduces their chances of conceiving a baby. However, unless the woman learns to watch for signs in her body that indicate the time of ovulation very precisely—for instance, keeping a chart of her body temperature—there is a strong chance of making a mistake.

A REST BETWEEN BABIES

A woman's body is designed in such a way that she is not likely to have another baby if she is still breastfeeding her last baby. The hormones that tell her body to produce milk also cause other messages to be sent to her ovaries so that no more egg cells are produced. The idea is that her body should not have to do too many things at once.

However, this method is not completely reliable.

CONTRACEPTION

Over the years people have invented artificial methods to prevent conception from taking place. These are called methods of contraception. They work in different ways.

The contraceptive pill contains chemicals that stop a woman's body from producing eggs. There is a 'mini' pill that makes the mucus of the cervix too thick for the sperms to get through.

Condoms used by men and diaphragms used by women are rubber barriers. They are used with a special cream to keep sperms and eggs from meeting. The condom is a protective sheath that fits over a man's penis. The diaphragm is slipped inside a woman's vagina so that it fits over the cervix.

There are also intrauterine devices which can be placed inside a woman's uterus. These are usually made of plastic with copper and silver wire around them. They stop a pregnancy developing.

None of these methods is 100 per cent successful.

Some religious groups, such as the Roman Catholic Church, forbid the use of artificial methods of contraception.

WHAT MAKES A FAMILY?

It takes two people to make a baby—a man and a woman. The Bible tells us that the father and the mother have an important role to play in supporting each other and bringing up their children.

In some countries a typical family consists only of the parents and children. In others, grandparents and aunts and uncles may all belong to one household. This extended family can provide even more support.

Families, like people, come in a variety of shapes and sizes. Some couples don't have children, but they are still a family. Some families adopt children who are in need of people to take care of them as they grow up. There are many reasons why some families have only one parent. It can still be a happy family, although the people in it will have to work harder to support each other. People outside the family can also provide lots of help and support.

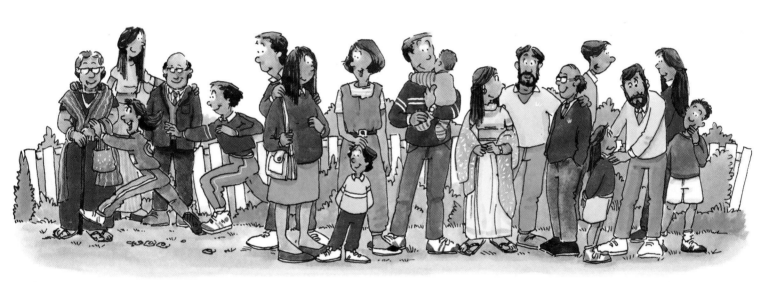

COUPLES WITHOUT KIDS

Some couples find that the woman does not become pregnant even though they have intercourse at the right time for many months. Sometimes doctors can find something in either the man's or the woman's body that needs to be set right. Meanwhile, the couple can have fun sharing the load of other people's children, even though they may continue to long for their own.

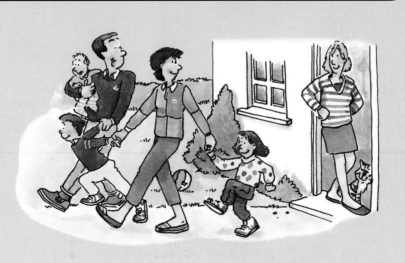

'TEST-TUBE BABIES'

In the last few years, doctors have also found ways to take sperms and use them to fertilize egg cells in a dish in the laboratory. The fertilized cell then starts to grow, and when it does it can be put inside the woman's uterus, where it can continue to develop in the usual way.

IMPORTANT QUESTIONS

Sexual intercourse is a very private act. It is meant to be so. But knowing how our bodies work, and where sex fits in, does not have to be a dark secret. It is important to talk to grown-ups you can trust if you have questions. Parents really want to help, and they can often give lots of useful information and advice. In other cases, a doctor or a teacher you can trust may be able to deal with your questions.

Even so, because some people feel that they can't talk about sex, you may be left with questions that you would like to ask but think that you have no one to answer them. Here are some of those questions—and some answers.

Q *Is masturbation OK?*

A It is quite natural to enjoy the pleasant sensation of touch, and touching the penis or the clitoris is enjoyable. It is meant to be, as part of making intercourse enjoyable. Self-stimulation is called masturbation. It can be used to help someone enjoy love-making with their partner. However, some people become addicted to it, and then they find they have to imagine all kinds of sexual situations to make it "work". These fantasies are not a good idea. Sexual excitement is to be shared with a loved and trusted partner, not used selfishly.

Q *Am I homosexual?*

A After puberty it is usual for boys to be attracted to girls and girls to boys. These relationships are called heterosexual, meaning that they involve people of two sexes. It is also quite usual for most people to admire people of the same sex and enjoy being in their company. However, when a relationship between two people of the same sex includes sexual attraction and the kind of kissing and body contact that usually occurs before sexual intercourse, then it is called homosexual.

Homosexual men are sometimes called gay, and homosexual women are called lesbians.

People do not know why some people are sexually attracted to others of the same sex. The Bible clearly teaches that it is wrong to take part in homosexual acts, just as it teaches that sexual intercourse is meant only to take place only between husband and wife. It expects all people to be in control of their behavior. However, God doesn't blame a person for being born with confused emotions, and neither should anyone else.

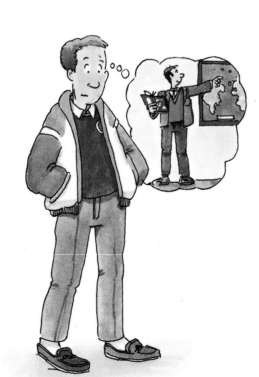

Q *What if a woman doesn't want to be pregnant?*

A There are all kinds of reasons why a woman might not want to be pregnant. It may be that her body is not strong enough to have a baby, and the strain of pregnancy could even kill her. It may be that she is not married to the father and has no plans to have a family.

There are medical ways of ending a pregnancy. If a pregnancy is stopped it is called an abortion. This is not the same as a spontaneous abortion, which happens naturally and carries less long-term risk to the woman's health. Of course, when a pregnancy is stopped the little life that is developing is ended.

Are there any reasons strong enough for not wanting a baby to justify ending it in this way? People today have many different opinions. One thing is certain: it is much better for a woman not to become pregnant if she does not want to have a baby.

Some religious groups, such as the Roman Catholic Church, forbid abortion.

Q *What is a virgin?*

A The word "virgin" simply means a person who has not had sexual intercourse. Both boys and girls can be called virgins.

Q *Can intercourse spread infection?*

A It certainly can. There are various illnesses that can be passed from one partner to the other by intercourse. Some of these can be treated fairly easily. Others can cause more serious problems and may result in the inability to have babies.

AIDS, or Acquired Immune Deficiency Syndrome, is the most serious disease spread by intercourse these days. It is caused by a virus known as HIV (Human Immuno-deficiency Virus) which is found in the body fluids of infected people. These fluids include saliva, semen, blood and urine. There is no known cure for AIDS.

Obviously, people who have only one partner—their husband or wife—are much less likely to have any of the infections that are spread by sexual intercourse.

Q *Can you catch AIDS just by being with someone who has it?*

A AIDS is not spread by everyday contact, such as shaking hands or simply hugging. People who have AIDS need their friends.

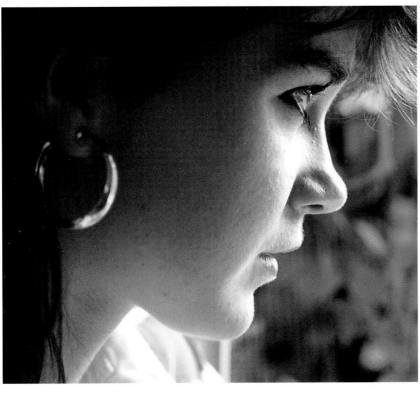

Q Is it OK to look at sexy magazines?

A A husband and wife are expected to enjoy the sight of each other's bodies. Within marriage, a naked body is meant to be exciting. Sexy magazines, books and videos, appeal to the same emotions. They are full of pictures of people with no clothes on doing sexy things. They are designed to give a bit of a thrill—a little taste of sex outside of marriage. That is a problem in itself. And who are the models in these materials? The men, women and children in these sexy poses are sometimes forced into this work, whether they like it or not. The industry that produces sexy materials exploits people in a horrible way.

Q Someone in my family keeps trying to treat me in a sexy way. What can I do?

A Anyone who tries to treat you as a sex object is abusing you. It might be quite slight, such as touching you in a way you don't like, or it might be as serious as sexual intercourse. No one has the right to treat you in this way: no one in your family, nor anyone in your school. It is against the law and it is wrong.

Too many young people suffer this type of abuse in silence. There are many people who want to help you, and you should go to them. It might be a doctor, a teacher at your school, or perhaps someone older whom you can trust. Tell them what is upsetting you simply and without making it seem better or worse than it really is.

You are not to blame for what is happening. God accepts you just as you are. You will be able to deal with the problem and get over the anger that you feel.

Q My friends tell sexy jokes, but I don't think they're funny. Am I missing something?

A People tell sexy jokes usually to show how brave and sophisticated they are when talking about sex. The reality is that most of them tell jokes about sex because they're too embarrassed to talk about it in a sensible way. Often the stories aren't funny at all. They may in fact be very cruel.

You're not missing anything except silliness.

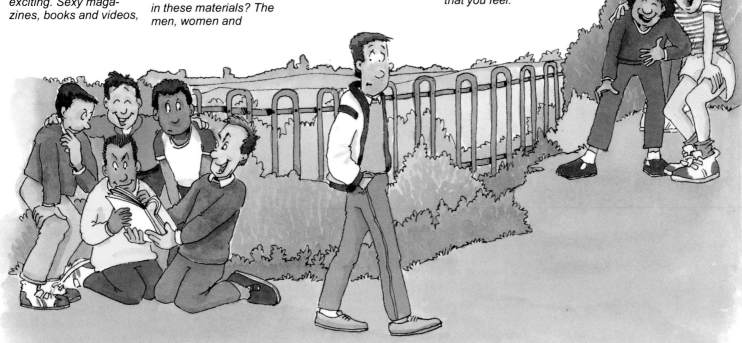

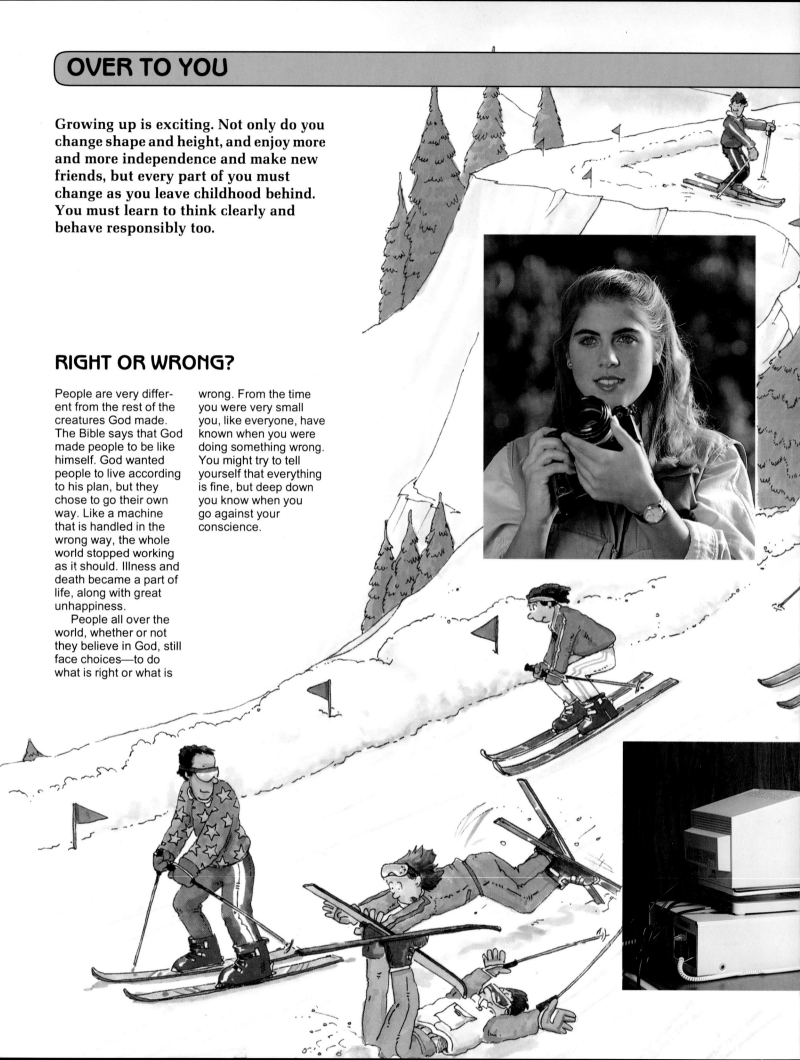

Growing up is exciting. Not only do you change shape and height, and enjoy more and more independence and make new friends, but every part of you must change as you leave childhood behind. You must learn to think clearly and behave responsibly too.

RIGHT OR WRONG?

People are very different from the rest of the creatures God made. The Bible says that God made people to be like himself. God wanted people to live according to his plan, but they chose to go their own way. Like a machine that is handled in the wrong way, the whole world stopped working as it should. Illness and death became a part of life, along with great unhappiness.

People all over the world, whether or not they believe in God, still face choices—to do what is right or what is wrong. From the time you were very small you, like everyone, have known when you were doing something wrong. You might try to tell yourself that everything is fine, but deep down you know when you go against your conscience.

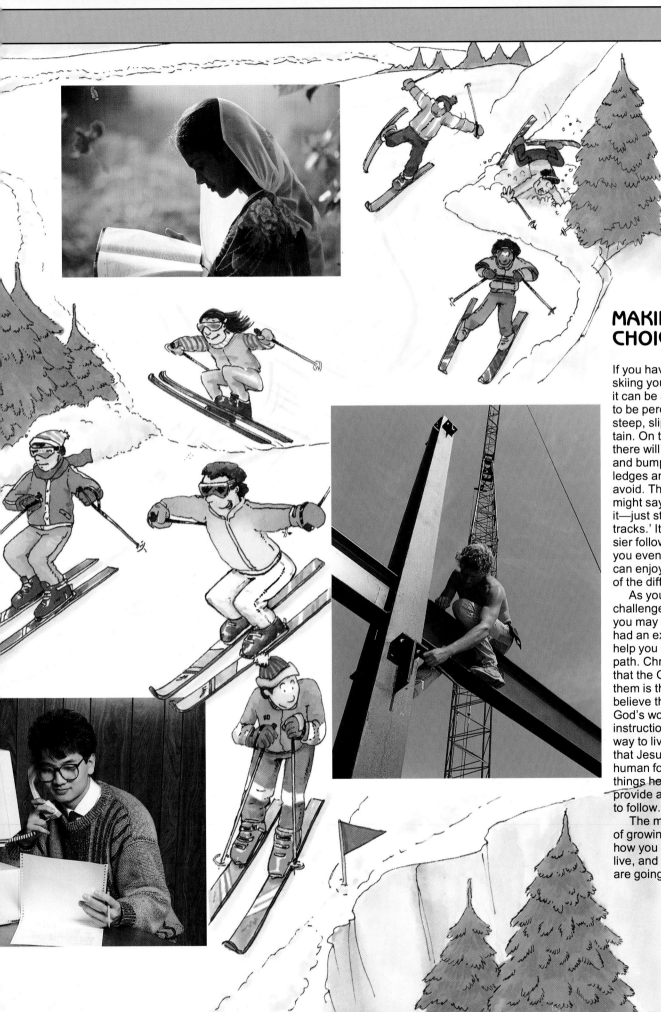

MAKING CHOICES

If you have ever been skiing you will know that it can be a bit frightening to be perched on top of a steep, slippery mountain. On the way down there will be icy patches and bumps, narrow ledges and trees to avoid. The instructor might say, 'You can do it—just stay in my tracks.' It is so much easier following the expert; you even find that you can enjoy the challenge of the difficult places!

As you go through the challenge of growing up, you may wish that you had an expert in living to help you stay on the right path. Christians believe that the God who made them is this expert. They believe that the Bible is God's word, containing instructions on the right way to live. They believe that Jesus was God in human form, and that the things he did and taught provide a model for them to follow.

The most serious part of growing up is deciding how you are going to live, and the choices you are going to make.

INDEX

**Answer to quiz on
spread 15: 25 Dec and
2 May**